Ophthalmological Considerations
in the Rehabilitation
of the Blind

Ophthalmological Considerations
in the Rehabilitation
of the Blind

By

CHARLES W. HOEHNE

*Assistant Director and Legal Counsel
for Texas State Commission for the Blind
Austin, Texas*

JOHN G. CULL, Ph.D.

*Professor of Clinical Counseling Psychology
Our Lady of the Lake University
San Antonio, Texas*

RICHARD E. HARDY, Ed.D.

*Chairman, Department of Rehabilitation Counseling
Virginia Commonwealth University
Richmond, Virginia*

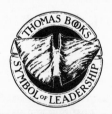

CHARLES C THOMAS • PUBLISHER
Springfield · Illinois · U.S.A.

Published and Distributed Throughout the World by
CHARLES C THOMAS • PUBLISHER
Bannerstone House
301-327 East Lawrence Avenue, Springfield, Illinois, U.S.A.

© *1980, by* CHARLES C THOMAS • PUBLISHER

ISBN 0-398-03812-0

Library of Congress Catalog Card Number: 79-11351

With THOMAS BOOKS *careful attention is given to all details of
manufacturing and design. It is the Publisher's desire to present books that
are satisfactory as to their physical qualities and artistic possibilities and
appropriate for their particular use.* THOMAS BOOKS *will be true to those
laws of quality that assure a good name and good will.*

Printed in the United States of America
V-R-2

Library of Congress Cataloging in Publication Data

Main entry under title:

Ophthalmological considerations in the rehabilitation of
the blind.

Includes index.
1. Blindness--Psychological aspects. 2. Blind--
Rehabilitation. 3. Physician and patient. 4. Ophthal-
mology. I. Hoehne, Charles W. II. Cull, John G.
III. Hardy, Richard E.
RE91.063   362.4'1   79-11351
ISBN 0-398-03812-0

*This book is dedicated to
one of the outstanding
leaders in the field
of the rehabilitation of the blind*

Douglas C. MacFarland, Ph.D.

CONTRIBUTORS

PAUL BACH-Y-RITA, M.D.: Professor, Department of Visual Sciences, School of Medical Sciences, University of the Pacific; Associate Director, Smith-Kettelwell Institute of Visual Sciences; Consultant on Sensory Aids for the National Eye Institute.

MARY K. BAUMAN: Director, Nevil Interagency Referral Service; Executive Secretary, Association for Education of the Visually Handicapped at the University of Pennsylvania; Chairman, Policy and Planning Board for Comprehensive Statewide Planning for Vocational Rehabilitation.

WARREN BLEDSOE: Principal Consultant to the Office for the Blind and Visually Handicapped, Rehabilitation Services Administration, Department of Health, Education and Welfare; Program Director, Department of Medicine Surgery for Blinded Veterans, Veterans Administration; Board Member, Maryland School for the Blind.

BEATRIX COBB, Ph.D.: Retired Horn Professor of Psychology and Former Director of Counselor Training, Department of Psychology, Texas Tech University; Head, Medical Psychology Section, University of Texas; Associate Professor, University of Texas Post-graduate School of Medicine.

CRISS COLE: District Judge, Harris County, Texas; University of Houston; Former state senator.

WILLIAM T. COPPAGE: Director, Virginia Commission for the Visually Handicapped; Assistant Director, Virginia Commission for the Visually Handicapped; Supervisor, Rehabilitation Evaluation and Training Program for the Blind (Virginia); Assistant Superintendent, Virginia

Workshop for the Blind.

FRANCES CRAWFORD: Rehabilitation Teaching Specialist, Bureau for the Visually Handicapped (Pennsylvania)

HAROLD CROSS, M.D., Ph.D.: Associate Professor of Ophthalmology and Surgery, University of Arizona College of Medicine.

JOHN G. CULL, Ph.D.: Professor of Clinical Counseling, Department of Psychology, Our Lady of the Lake University of San Antonio. Formerly, Director, Regional Continuing Education Program and Professor of Rehabilitation Counseling, Department of Rehabilitation Counseling, Virginia Commonwealth University, Fishersville, Virginia; Rehabilitation Counselor, Texas Rehabilitation Commission and Texas State Commission for the Blind; Assistant Commissioner (Director of Research and Program Development), Virginia State Department of Vocational Rehabilitation; Technical Consultant, Rehabilitation Services Administration, United States Department of Health, Education, and Welfare, Washington, D. C.

WILLIAM F. GALLAGHER: Director, Program Planning Department, American Foundation for the Blind; Director of Rehabilitation, New York Association for the Blind (lighthouse); Director, Greater Pittsburgh Guild for the Blind; Chief of Professional Services, Catholic Guild for the Blind (Boston).

CHARLES GALLOZZI: Assistant Chief, Division for the Blind and Visually Handicapped, Library of Congress; Chief, Library for the Blind (Philadelphia).

RICHARD E. HARDY, Ed.D.: Chairman, Department of Rehabilitation Counseling, Virginia Commonwealth University, Richmond, Virginia; Technical Consultant, United States Department of Health, Education, and Welfare, Rehabilitation Services Administration, Washington, D. C. Formerly, Rehabilitation Counselor in Virginia; Rehabilitation Advisor, Rehabilitation Services Administration, United States Department of Health, Education, and Welfare, Washington, D. C.; former Chief

Psychologist and Supervisor of Professional Training, South Carolina Department of Rehabilitation; member of the South Carolina State Board of Examiners in Psychology.

WILLIAM M. HART, Ph.D., M.D.: Professor and Chairman, Department of Ophthalmology, University of Missouri, Columbia, Missouri; Executive Director, Eye Research Foundation of Missouri.

CHARLES W. HOEHNE: Assistant Director and Legal Counsel for Texas State Commission for the Blind.

RICHARD E. HOOVER, M.D.: Assistant Professor in Ophthalmology, Johns Hopkins School of Medicine; Chief of Ophthalmology, Greater Baltimore Medical Center.

ARTHUR H. KEENEY, M.D.: Dean and Professor of Ophthalmology, University of Louisville School of Medicine; Director of Ophthalmic Research and Associate Professor of Ophthalmology, University of Pennsylvania.

JOSEPH KOHN: Director, New Jersey State Commission for the Blind and Visually Impaired; Chairman, Board of Trustees, Eye Institute of New Jersey.

PAYTON KOLB, M.D.: Consultant, Arkansas Enterprises for the Blind; Director, Research and Education, State Hospital, Little Rock; Clinical Professor of Psychiatry, University of Arkansas Medical Center.

KATHY F. LEVINSON, M.S. (RC): Formerly area director for the American Cancer Society in Boston; medical social worker at the Medical College of Virginia and Virginia Commonwealth University.

HARRY J. LINK: Specialist in Placement and Employment, Program Development Division, American Foundation for the Blind.

DOUGLAS C. MACFARLAND, Ph.D.: Director, Office for the Blind and Visually Handicapped, Rehabilitation Services Administration, Department of Health, Education, and Welfare; Director, Virginia Commission for the Visually Handicapped; Vocational Counselor and Supervisor, Delaware Commission for the Blind.

LORRAINE H. MARCHI: Founder and Executive Director, National Association for Visually Handicapped; Past Chairman of the Board, Langley Porter Neuropsychiatric Institute, University of California Medical Center.

BENJAMIN MILDER, M.D.: Associate Professor of Clinical Ophthalmology, Department of Ophthalmology, Washington University School of Medicine.

JAMES L. MIMS, JR., M.D.: Clinical Professor of Ophthalmology, University of Texas Medical School in San Antonio.

FRANK L. MYERS, M.D.: Assistant Clinical Professor of Ophthalmology, University of Wisconsin.

HEDWIG OSWALD, M.S.: Director, Selective Placement Programs, United States Civil Service Commission; Program Manager, Selective Placement Programs; Project Coordinator, Federal Employment of the Mentally Retarded.

BURT L. RISLEY: Executive Director, Texas State Commission for the Blind; Past President, Texas Chapter, American Association of Workers for the Blind.

LOUIS H. RIVES, JR.: Director, Health and Social Services Division, Office of Civil Rights; Chief, Social Welfare and Related Programs Division, Office of Civil Rights; Special Assistant to the Commissioner of Vocational Rehabilitation, Department of Health, Education, and Welfare; Past President, American Association of Workers for the Blind.

PREFACE

HISTORICALLY, cultures up to and including our own have been concerned and somewhat sensitized regarding the needs of blind and visually handicapped individuals. Since the impact of loss of vision is so severe, it has long been recognized that no one discipline or professional practitioner has the expertise or background to adequately meet even the more evident needs of this group. Therefore it is widely accepted that a team effort is required. Nevertheless this is the first definitive text on the interfacing or joint efforts that should be mounted by ophthalmology and vocational rehabilitation to substantially improve the rehabilitation potential of this segment of our population.

This book is written by professional practitioners in both fields and as such is characterized by its pragmatism. This text presents concepts that may be readily implemented in service programs and appear to have a high probability of increasing the level of services to the visually impaired. We feel this group of professional practitioners should be commended for this contribution to the professional literature.

John G. Cull
Richard E. Hardy

CONTENTS

Ophthalmological Considerations
in the Rehabilitation
of the Blind

CHAPTER 1

CRISES IN INSTITUTIONS: OPHTHALMOLOGY AND REHABILITATION ARE NOT IMMUNE

CRISS COLE

THE era in which we now live is one in which many institutions are under attack, being challenged, and unendingly questioned. Few, if any, of our traditional institutions escape being challenged or threatened. Some of this may be necessary and even healthy. Much of it, however, seems to be going on simply because it is popular or fashionable.

Few institutions are immune from crisis, and some may not successfully withstand the problems with which they are now attempting to deal.

An almost unprecedented rate of inflation, coupled with tight money and a scarcity of items as basic as food or gasoline, causes many of this country's strongest economic institutions to be faced with a crisis of proportions we have not seen since the Great Depression.

Changing values and life styles present some of our churches with declining memberships and serious problems of financial solvency.

Education is under attack from all directions — students resent being graduated without marketable skills; taxpayers revolt in reaction to growing property tax burdens; and teachers start forming unions out of sheer frustration and desperation.

The reformers attack our traditional system of conducting political campaigns and elections, noting that the high costs of television and advertising make it inappropriate to talk about "free elections" in the United States. The institution of the presidency is subjected to the most serious challenge ever in the life of this nation.

Our legal institutions are not immune to challenge and crisis. If there is some sort of Rip Van Winkle in the legal profession who received his license twenty years ago and who has since been sleeping, he will find when he awakes that he is obsolete because of not having kept up with all of the landmark changes the legal profession has had to absorb during the past several years.

Neither do I think that any of you would suggest that ophthalmology and rehabilitation are immune to crisis. Those of you who represent medicine will not find it necessary for me to discuss the many problems you confront from so many directions. Those of you who represent rehabilitation, one of the oldest and most successful federal grant - in - aid programs ever established in the United States, have seen legislation for which state agencies for the blind have been working for years unanimously enacted by the Congress, subjected to two vetoes, and those vetoes sustained.

The question is not whether some of the more time-honored institutions of this nation are undergoing crisis — that is self-evident.

The salient questions are why are these continuing crises being experienced, what can we do to resolve those problems, and what are the realistic prospects of some of our more venerable institutions — including medicine as it has traditionally been practiced and rehabilitation services as they historically have been conducted — withstanding the major challenges which now confront them?

I think that there are a number of reasons for these continuing challenges. Some of these reasons are good, some are valid, and some are without merit. I am confident that in virtually every instance in which crisis exists because of a bona fide necessity to respond more effectively to human needs, rehabilitation and ophthamology are going to meet the challenge successfully.

The problem which confronts so many institutions today is that, on the one hand, things are becoming so much more complicated than ever before and, on the other hand, those whom the institutions serve are expecting so much more than ever before, to the extent that totally unrealistic demands are sometimes made.

All of us are confronted with an explosion of technical information. A year now brings more scientific and technical developments than we once had in a decade. This is true of virtually every professional field and certainly is not restricted to ophthalmology or rehabilitation. The sheer bulk of these new developments is so massive it is impossible for any one professional to absorb all of it.

So we start to specialize, and then we start to subspecialize. In law, it is no longer enough for an attorney to specialize in the tax field; today, there are people who are making their entire careers in one very narrow area of the entire tax field, such as handling tax-sheltered retirement programs.

There are fewer and fewer family doctors around and an increasing number of specialists. The same thing is true in rehabilitation. There are counselors who specialize in evaluation, some who specialize in motivating clients and helping them to understand blindness, others who specialize in vocational placement, and still others who work primarily as managers of services provided through a broad variety of resources. There are rehabilitation teachers who specialize in teaching personal adjustment skill to clients who are simply blind, while other rehabilitation teachers work with multiply-handicapped cases, and still others specialize in working with geriatric cases. Therapists with all sorts of subspecialties are utilized at rehabilitation centers which offer selected programs designed for clients who fit into various categories. New occupational titles are constantly being developed to describe some of the innovative services being provided by new breeds of workers who are graduating from training programs which did not exist five or ten years ago.

In the main, this is good. It reflects that we are fortunate enough to have increased sophistication. It shows that we have a greater capacity to meet human needs more adequately.

But I sometimes wonder if all of these changes do not also have disadvantages. I sometimes wonder if all of this impetus toward specialization and subspecialization does not have a natural tendency to force us to become highly preoccupied with final professional points, to the extent that we sometimes lose perspective and lose sight of the total human problems of the people for whom all of this specialization and subspecialization presumably exists.

This explosion in scientific and technical knowledge is not something that occurs in a vacuum or in isolation. It is an informational explosion that is accompanied by an equally important and perhaps even more significant explosive element — the revolutionary, broadening expectations which people have in terms of the institutions which they feel should exist to serve people.

These days people expect more and they demand more — *and when they do not perceive that performance is commensurate to their expectations, institutions are in trouble.* When you get right down to the final analysis, is this not why rehabilitation has been having difficulty with its legislation, its new administrative regulations, and its appropriations? Is this not why medicine must wrestle with at least some of the challenges which presently confront the profession?

Some of these expectations most certainly are unrealistic. Are some of these expectations, however, totally unreasonable?

If one holds a license to practice law, if one has been licensed to practice medicine, if one earns his living through the comparative security of employment on a state or federal payroll, or if one is involved with some sort of program enjoying nonprofit tax status, then people tend to see the person as being somehow in a favored, special, or privileged position.

In a very real sense, those of us who do happen to occupy such positions are in fact endowed with a somewhat favored, special, or privileged status. These licenses, claims to public resources, or tax-exempt statuses do in fact give us a bit of an edge over others. With this edge, there necessarily is a higher degree of *accountability*.

What, exactly, is it to which we are to be held accountable? I submit that it is neither fair nor reasonable for any professional in any specialized field to be held accountable for anything for which he does not profess to have special credentials by reason of his training, experience, or natural abilities. None of us, however extraordinarily capable or totally committed or entirely hard-working, have or profess to possess the talent, capacities, or resources for resolving all of the problems of the increasingly complicated world in which we must live.

Nor do I think that in holding us or the institutions we represent accountable for performance, any fair-minded person asks or expects that we be able to solve all of the problems of the world.

What is expected, in my judgment, is a continuing consciousness of the fact that this increasingly complex world in which we live is a world made up of not fine professional points, not simply scientific discoveries, not merely technical innovations, not just specialties and subspecialties but of *people*. It is, in fact, for people that all of these scientific discoveries, technical innovations, specialties, and subspecialties exist. I suggest to you that if we keep this point foremost in our minds, then none of us nor any of the institutions we represent are very likely to get into any serious trouble.

We cannot be all things to all people; but we can be people helping people to be people. If we can accomplish this while bringing to bear the highest and best of the special skills, knowledge, and expertise we or the institutions we represent might have, then I think this is all that can, should, or will be expected of us.

Today it is no longer sufficient, if it ever was, for a lawyer simply to be highly learned in the law. The lawyer who is simply highly learned in the law but not sensitive to the total human needs of his client is not adequate as an individual — and probably will not be regarded as an adequate attorney by many of his clients.

By the same token, the physician who is simply highly skilled in the practice of medicine is no longer regarded, if he ever was, as adequately equipped to meet the more basic expectations his patients have of him.

The rehabilitation worker for the blind who is highly trained and experienced in conducting some selective phase of rehabili-

tation services — counseling, guidance, skills training, placement, or whatever — is also not going to be able to satisfy the
expectations of his clients if that worker is unable to recognize
and appreciate all of the problems, direct and indirect, obvious
or subtle, that impinge upon the client and retard the client's
ability to function as an adequate, effective human being.

Institutional crisis is, essentially, the accumulation of isolated and individualistic instances of personal inadequacy, in-
sensitivity, or indifference. Jurisprudence does not in the
abstract bring law into public disrepute, but rather the specific
and concrete acts of individual lawyers — their errors and
omissions — bring law into occasional disrepute. I am in-
clined to believe that the same is true with medicine and rehabilitation.

It follows, then, that the accountability which attaches to
institutions is in reality an extension of the personal accountability which attaches to each of us who are a part of, involved
with, and make up various institutions.

It does not, however, follow that institutions which are so
greatly challenged today will in time perish unless we are individually able to resolve personally all of the problems of each
of the persons we are called upon to serve.

It is enough, I think, if we each do the best that we can,
maintaining a keen sensitivity to the total problems of those
whom we serve, a willingness to recognize our own personal
inabilities to resolve all of their varied problems, and the capacity to turn to and reach out for others to assist us in treating
problems which may be beyond our own professional capacities.

This is basically what this book is all about — to impart a
better idea of what each of these professions (medicine and
rehabilitation) now has to offer Americans who are blind or in
danger of becoming blind, and to develop mechanisms to assure that respective skills, knowledge, and resources are
brought into play in a more coordinated manner, so that the
benefits of these two professions respectively can be enhanced
in a manner which should by far exceed the enhancement
which can be achieved through any dozen scientific or technical
breakthroughs in either field.

I think this book is worthy of emulation in many fields beyond the field of services to the blind and visually handicapped. I most certainly hope that the model which is being provided will commend itself to many other professions involved in services to people.

How appropriate it is that those who are so vitally involved in serving the blind and visually handicapped should once more be providing the example to other professions and to other fields. This, after all, is a long and proud tradition.

Ophthalmological surgery, I have been told by some authorities, began over 2000 years ago when an Egyptian removed cataracts for the first time — using a sliver of a cane reed for his scalpel.

Work for the blind, it has been said, dates back at least as far as that first cataract extraction. Throughout the history of work for the blind, there has been a constant and consistent theme: those who were involved in this work provided the innovation, the example, and the model and others came along and adapted this to other fields. I think there exists an opportunity for renewing this historic cycle.

Those who are contributing to this text as leading representatives of ophthalmology and rehabilitation can fire a shot which will one day be heard throughout the broad field of services to people.

I urge you who read this book to fire such shots and to be on target. I also urge you to remember that the reverberation will not be determined only by what you do, but even more by what you do cooperatively as the most eminent representatives of two old and honorable institutions. If what you are attempting to accomplish is substantially accomplished, your efforts will have been more than worthwhile solely because of the benefits which will accrue to blind and visually handicapped Americans. If you are successful, then inevitably what you accomplish will find itself extended to other groups who may find themselves in distressed circumstances. I can foresee the day when cooperative efforts of this type will be fashionable and effective in providing a similar type of interdisciplinary exchange and a basis for joint planning among other professions in other areas. I can see lawyers who work primarily in the representation of persons injured in accidents meeting with orthopedic surgeons, the heads of general rehabilitation programs meeting with cardiologists for the benefit of victims of strokes or heart attacks, and numerous other possibilities of cooperative effort.

More importantly, I can very readily appreciate the implications this holds for the people for whom institutions or professions exist.

Accordingly, I regard it as a high honor to have been invited to contribute this introductory chapter.

References and Suggested Readings

1. Bloom, Bernard L.: Human accountability in a community mental health center: Report of an automated system. *Community Ment Health J, 8* (4):251-260, 1972.

2. *Critical issues involved in rehabilitation of the severely handicapped.* Report of the study group, First Institute on Rehabilitation Issues, April 15-17, 1974, Denver, Colorado. Hot Springs, Arkansas, Arkansas Rehabilitation Research and Training Center, University of Arkansas, April 1974.

3. Harrington, John T.: Directions in medical curriculum. *The Mission of the University of Texas Health Science Center at San Antonio, 3* (1):2-4, Spring 1976.

4. Laski, Frank: Civil rights victories for the handicapped. *Social and Rehabilitation Record, 1* :15-20, 1974.

5. MacFarland, Douglas C.: International and national projects on blindness. In Hardy, Richard E. and Cull, John G. (Eds.): *Social and Rehabilitation Services for the Blind.* Springfield, Thomas, 1972, pp. 88-99.

6. Muthard, J. E. and Salamone, P. R.: The roles and functions of the rehabilitation counselor. *Rehabilitation Counseling Bulletin (Special Issue), 13* (1-SP):18-168, 1969.

7. *Papers on the national health guidelines: Baselines for setting health goals and standards.* HEW, Public Health Service, Health Resources Administration, Publication No. (HRA), 76-640. Washington, D. C., Govt Print Office, September 1976.

8. *Planning services for the blind for the decade of the '70's.* Final report of a conference held in Hazelwood, Missouri, March 25 — 28, 1973. With support from HEW, Rehabilitation Services Administration, Social and Rehabilitation Services.

9. Rubin, Stanford E. (Ed.): *Studies on the evaluation of state vocational rehabilitation agency programs: A summary report.* Research Report No. 889. Arkansas Rehabilitation Research and Training Center, September 1975.

CHAPTER 2

REHABILITATION'S EVOLVING PERCEPTION OF A BROADENED MISSION

DOUGLAS C. MACFARLAND

VOCATIONAL rehabilitation is by no means a new concept. In fact, the state-federal program will celebrate its sixtieth anniversary in 1980. The fundamental principles of rehabilitation, however, have been practiced in work for the blind for a much longer period of time. The basic roots in this country go back to the early nineteenth century. Unfortunately, the concept of rehabilitating the severely disabled, including the blind, was not officially incorporated into our law until 1943 with the passage of the Barden-LaFollette Act, Public Law No. 113. The late start meant that we had to do a great deal of work in order to move the program to the competitive position it now holds. Of course, a tremendous impetus was given to Public Law No. 113 because of its fortuitous passage during World War II when jobs were plentiful and the resistance to employing a severely disabled person was minimal.

For comparative purposes, I think it would be interesting to note the changes that have taken place since the early years of the Barden-LaFollette Act. At the end of 1943, there were less than 1,000 blind and severely visually impaired rehabilitated into employment. Figures for 1975 show an increase to 28,700. In the early years, the emphasis was centered on industrial jobs, vending stand operations, and sheltered workshop employment. With the growth of the program, employment opportunities expanded along with more sophisticated techniques for training blind and severely visually impaired persons to cope with loss of vision in the performance of their jobs and normal social activities. As others will indicate in later chapters, in

12

1954 the Vocational Rehabilitation Act was expanded to include research and training activities. The incorporation of training programs for professionals in the field and funding for research activities added immeasurably to the possibilities for reducing the time lag in coping with many of the needs and providing adequate personnel necessary to meet many of the challenges in our field in a much shorter period of time than might otherwise have been possible.

Let me hasten to add that we have by no means reached our ultimate goal of a total service delivery system for all blind and severely visually impaired persons. We can, however, look with a good deal of pride at what has happened in the last four decades. In the early forties, as I indicated at the outset, employment for the blind consisted of vending stand operations, jobs in industry, and employment in sheltered workshops. There were, of course, exceptions, but these were considered unusual. Today, employment opportunities for blind persons are enormously expanded. There are thousands of different jobs that are feasible for blind persons, many that would have been considered highly impractical even by most of our counselors in the late fifties — physicists, engineers, radio and TV technicians, computer programming (including the more sophisticated jobs in systems analysis), meteorologists, psychiatrists, and teachers of sighted children in the public school system to mention a few. Others will discuss in later chapters the more exotic results of research in medicine, hardware, and new instructional techniques.

I should like to cover briefly what I consider the fundamentals of rehabilitation. The basic model is what some of us call the "rehabilitation cycle" consisting of seven steps.

1. *Diagnostic Evaluation* — Including medical and specialty examinations; psychological testing; family, recreational, educational, and vocational experience; and initial counseling.

2. *Physical Restoration* — Which is of paramount importance before basic training begins. Can the applicant be restored to his optimum physical condition? This means, of course, treatment necessary to improve or stabilize any health problems that might be apparent. In the case of the blind or

visually impaired person, this of course would mean medical eye treatment and surgery. While we are firmly committed to providing the high quality services required to help a blind or visually impaired person achieve his maximum vocational potential, there is no question that the best rehabilitation possible is the improvement or restoration of sight.

3. *Counseling* — Pulling together all the information obtained and working very closely with the client, developing the most suitable job objective and an agreed-upon plan for attaining the goal.

4. *Prevocational or Adjustment Training* — For the visually impaired person this means provision of services that will assist the individual insofar as possible to cope with the problems of his disability and to return to a place of dignity in society and the working world.

5. *Training* — In accordance with the vocational rehabilitation plan developed, obtain the necessary training to compete favorably in the occupation of the individual's choice. Training may range from dishwasher to college professor and includes just about everything in between.

6. *Placement* — Here one provides all assistance necessary to effect appropriate placement. Here too is a wide variety of activities ranging from direct contact with employers to helping the skilled worker and university-trained person to develop job resumes, make appointments, and develop necessary public relations in the case of individuals opening businesses or entering professions.

7. *Post-employment and Follow-up Services* — Are provided to make certain that the individual is competing with his peers and to assist with any problems that may arise. This may include on-the-job counseling, assistance with family problems, and the purchase of newly-developed equipment that will make the individual more competitive.

The most unique cluster of services provided in the rehabilitation cycle are those usually offered at a rehabilitation adjustment center for the blind. Here is where the blind person learns the special techniques that must be mastered in order to become socially and vocationally integrated — mobility skills (independent travel with the use of a cane or dog guide), activities of daily living, communications skills, the use of aids and appliances, and many other techniques that will be described in detail throughout the book.

Without successful mastery of these skills, total rehabilitation would become extremely difficult, if not impossible. As we have achieved greater success in vocational rehabilitation, the field has had an opportunity to assess the more difficult problems facing it and to mobilize professional resources to work toward their solution.

During the past few years, the rehabilitative techniques that were so useful for the young and middle-aged adult have begun to be applied to the older blind person, not for vocational achievement but to help such individuals attain the highest status of independent living possible. Although the work is essential, funds for such purposes have been extremely scarce.

We now have a few centers for specialized geriatric rehabilitation of the blind, but they can handle only a trickle of the thousands that apparently need the service. New social security legislation eventually will make funds available to expand services to the older blind. The methods used will be those pioneered by the rehabilitation movement.

A second area that is now receiving a modicum of attention involves the problems encountered by the multiply-handicapped blind client. Until recently, very little was done for these individuals. Due in part at least to vastly improved medical care, many more blind persons who have one or more major disabling conditions in addition to their blindness are applying for and receiving services.

Studies show that we can expect this number to increase substantially in the coming years. One study, conducted by Dr. Lowenfeld a few years ago of school-age blind children in California, indicated that more than 50 percent of the children investigated were suffering from severe disabilities in addition to blindness. This trend is evident in other states as well as California and certainly sounds a warning for all of us who will be providing rehabilitation services for these children in the next ten years.

A third area which has been neglected for much too long but is now getting some attention concerns the adjustment of the partially-sighted client. Individuals who had some residual vision heretofore were not considered good candidates for rehabilitation adjustment training. There is abundant evidence now, however, which indicates that special techniques can be devised and may be taught to the client with severe visual limitations in order to help him make maximum use of his remaining sight and to recognize limitations and work within them.

Our slow starts in the foregoing areas are mainly the results of inadequate funding and the desire to do the best job for the greatest number of individuals. With the passage of the Rehabilitation Act of 1973, Congress and the Administration have recognized the nature of the problem and hopefully the concomitant costs. At any rate, the law clearly mandates us to focus on the severely disabled client; this does not mean to the neglect of other disability groups, but highlights the necessity for setting priorities. The act also recognizes, and this for the first time in its more than fifty years of history, the need for rehabilitative services to certain groups who may not have a vocational orientation. This is specifically cited in Section 304, Special Projects. A small amount of money was appropriated this year for spinal cord injury centers and for projects with the underachieving deaf and older blind. In the case of the older blind, congressional testimony clearly indicated that these services need not be tied to a vocational objective.

The same section dealing with special projects appropriated construction money and operational funds for the National Center for Deaf-Blind Youths and Adults — a model facility to offer rehabilitation services to the most severely disabled deaf-blind persons in the country. The center also provides training for personnel who will, in turn, work in state and private facilities to provide rehabilitation services to those deaf-blind persons who can be assisted in their community. In addition, the center will conduct a national program of research, developing hardware and special techniques that will assist in minimizing the catastrophic effects of deaf-blindness and help these individuals achieve their rightful place in society.

Although the act fell short of including support for the many prevention of blindness programs that are now being conducted by state agencies throughout the country, it is my contention that the time has arrived for considerable expansion of these vital services. Even without specificity in project grants, a good deal of support for prevention activities can be made available through regular grant support. With careful planning these services can be expanded substantially through the expeditious use of medicaid, medicare, and social service funds.

This, then, is a brief outline of the evolution of rehabilitation aspects of work for the blind. We can be justifiably proud of the giant strides that have been taken in the past three decades and there is little need to apologize for our shortcomings, so long as we recognize that the few steps which we have taken are merely the beginning of the race.

The broadened mission of rehabilitation for the blind and severely visually impaired can be summed up in a very few words. For the multidisciplinary professionals, it means redoubling our efforts so that, in the lifetime of some of us, we will achieve total services for all who desire and can profit from them; for our partners who are engaged in ophthalmology it means a renewed dedication to work for the goal which has so often been articulated — the prevention of 50 percent of the blindness which is now extant in the country and the improved care of those for whom severe visual limitation of total blindness is an irreversible fact of life.

References

Lowenfeld, Berthold: *Multi-handicapped Blind Children in California.* Sacramento, California State Department of Education, Division of Special Services, 1968.

United States Congress: Barden-LaFollette Act, 78th Congress, Public Law No. 113. Washington, D. C., U. S. Govt Print Office, 1943.

United States Congress: Vocational Rehabilitation Act Amendments, 93rd Congress, 2nd session, S Doc No. 2759, Public Law No. 565.

Washington, D. C., U. S. Govt Print Office, 1954.
United States Congress: Rehabilitation Act Amendments, 93rd Congress, Public Law No. 93-112. Washington, D. C., U. S. Govt Print Office, 1973.

CHAPTER 3

CURRENT OPHTHALMIC ADVANCES IN THE PREVENTION OF BLINDNESS AND RESTORATION OF SIGHT

ARTHUR H. KEENEY

"To cure sometimes, to relieve frequently, to comfort always."
Anonymous, 15th Century

OPHTHALMOLOGY has made measurable strides of advancement in recent years. This advancement may be categorized under four headings: (I) Diagnostic Advances, (II) Therapeutic Advances, (III) Prognostic Advances, and (IV) Research Progress.

Diagnostic Advances

There are recent parallel advances both in knowledge of ocular disease and in instrumentation.

Disease Correlations

Variations and correlations in diseases components, though probably always to be incompletely understood, have come to markedly improved understanding in recent years. For example, it has become clear that sharp reduction of the pressure inside a glaucomatous eye, while desirably sought to protect the optic nerve from blinding inroads of glaucoma, may distinctly worsen retinal problems if the patient is a diabetic. Thus, we should tolerate somewhat higher intraocular pressures bordering the glaucomatous range for the diabetic than for the nondiabetic patient. Similarly, abrupt reductions in general or systemic blood pressure have been known to worsen

19

the eye's tolerance to moderate glaucoma. Thus a small degree of high blood pressure may help the needed pumping of arterial blood into the eye when increased intraocular pressure of glaucoma creates resistance to arterial access. Transient obscuration of vision (transient ischemic attacks) in one eye now are clearly understood to be early warning signs of obstruction in the major carotid artery on the same side of the neck. Prompt vascular surgery in the neck may both salvage vision and prevent a likely subsequent stroke afflicting the opposite side of the body.

Newly isolated infectious agents attacking both the cornea and the interior of the eye have been found recently both among fungi and viruses. These specific identifications, as the recent isolation of North American blastomycosis from an inflammed cornea, make possible highly specific treatment. The rapid development of new antibiotics from modern pharmaceutical research now enables the ophthalmologist to effectively counter both familiar bacteria which develop antibiotic resistances and unfamiliar pathogens which may invade the eye from other parts of the body or other animal reservoirs.

Instrumentation

Broad improvements in diagnostic instruments in the past few years enable the ophthalmologist now to approach an optimal number of diagnostic procedures in minimum time for conservation of patient energy and effort. This reduces formerly fatiguing examinations and obtains more valid information for the examiner.

Refinements in the indirect ophthalmoscope, the slit lamp microscope and the contact lens gonioscope now afford the ophthalmologist direct and extensive visualization of the previously obscured, far-peripheral retina, allowing him to see stereoscopically the early loss of optic nerve head fibers which should support the vital arteries needed to nourish the optic nerve in glaucoma — the "overpass" phenomenon described by George Link Spaeth, M.D., of Wills Eye Hospital — and to see and to manipulate minute aspects of the outflow chamber angle in the glaucomatous eye.

Fluorescent differentiation of minute arteries from veins and the identification of leaking areas in and deep to the retina by intravenous injection of fluroescein dye and timed photography of its flow through the vessels of the retina have now become commonplace. This greatly augments direct visual inspection and pinpoints previously obscure vascular failures inside the eye.

Ultrasound — like sonar to the fisherman seeking schools of fish in deep water or to the pilot probing water depth under his craft — now gives diagnostic tissue echoes localizing retinal detachments, hidden foreign bodies, and tumors deep in the eye. Ultrasound has become to soft tissue an equivalent of x-rays for the study of boney tissues. Only since 1973 has it been possible to visualize swelling of the optic nerve behind the eyeball by the widened and reduplicated contour of the nerve (Coleman's sign) seen in B-scan or two-dimensional echograms. Previously, diagnosis in this area had to be made by exclusion of more obvious diseases and then a *presumptive* diagnosis made, if nothing else of significance was left.

X-ray techniques to find small tumors, bone fragments, or foreign bodies in and behind the eye have been greatly improved by the slicing or lamellar technique producing successive views at specific depths through and behind the eye. Also in the past few years, xeroradiograms have greatly increased the latitude of film resolution, revealing elements of both high and low density on the same x-ray exposure. Also since 1973 the introduction of EMI scan and CAT scan has afforded enormously refined identification of minute masses or tumors in the optic nerve or within individual extraocular muscles.

Fiberoptics now make possible completely cool and painless delivery of high intensity light to transilluminate the eye and lids in search for tumors or radiolucent foreign bodies. Earlier incandescent lamps generated too much heat for tolerance by the ocular tissue. For more intense direct illumination, minature halogen bulbs offer greatly improved visualization and differentiation.

Electrodiagnostic analysis of minute currents in the retina

cells (electroretinogram) and in the light trapping pigment epithelium which backs the retina (electro-oculogram) give new objective information concerning actual functions and even impending damage in these tissues.

Foreign body localizers with improved electronics such as the Bronson-Turner localizer or the earlier Roper-Hall-Moon have increased sensitivity and are undisturbed by the earth's gravity. These enable ophthalmic surgeons to find unsuspected and damaging particles hidden within and around the injured eye.

Therapeutic Advances

Classical and long-established theoretical principles of optically compensated or aspheric lens surfaces recently have been translated at a practical production level into truly "wide field" lenses for postoperative cataract patients and into similarly improved proximal magnifying devices for low-vision aids. The concept of "minimum effective diameter" has been put into mass production by Robert C. Welsh of Miami, Florida, so that the previous, lens-inducted restrictions of field in high-powered lenses have been greatly reduced. Some producers, however, still seek compensation for optical abberations by using differences in radii of curvature of the two sides of a spherically ground lens (e.g. "crossed lenses" with a ratio of 1:6 for curvature of the two faces of the lens). Far finer resolution and image quality are achieved by precision casting of truly aspheric lenses.

Similarly, nineteenth century Fresnel principles of lens design by large numbers of contiguous prism angles make possible cheap and thin plastic magnifier sheets of high power and large area.

Distinctly improved understanding of cellular responses to and the complications of medicines now yield a highly efficient nonsurgical treatment for most patients with open-angle glaucoma. This was formerly called chronic simple or noncongestive glaucoma but now requires surgical drainage or filtration operations only when maximal medical treatment is inadequate. Essentially all cases of glaucoma can be brought under control if treatment is begun early and if the glaucoma is not a secondary complication of other precipitating diseases such as ocular tumor or obstruction of the outflow veins from the eye.

Surgical treatment of glaucoma has been reapproached recently by several new procedures to open the outflow filtration meshwork. One procedure, trabeculotomy, excises a segment of the drainage meshwork; this yields a tissue specimen for fundamental study and analysis both by light and by the greater magnification of electron microscopy. Surgical results in acute angle closure or narrow angle glaucoma by present techniques of iridectomy are generally immediately effective and sustained in their duration. Salvage by surgery (goniotomy and trabeculotomy) in early congenital glaucoma has improved, going from near total failure to a success rate of 50 to 60 percent when operated upon early in life. These results, however, are still grossly inferior to either medical or surgical expectations in adult onset glaucoma. Increasing genetic awareness makes earlier diagnosis and treatment much more frequent in affected families.

Refinement and miniaturization of surgical equipment now permits microsurgery under operating microscopes which afford critically detailed assessment of each anatomical component of the eye. Ocular surgeons have long operated with loups which give two- or three-fold magnification, but this is now extended to ten-fold with foot-operated and ceiling-suspended surgical microscopes.

Fine sutures producing almost no tissue reaction also have been facilitated and some of these, no thicker than three blood cells (21 mica), require modest microscopic magnification to be seen. This permits, unlike the older incisional drainage operations (cyclodialysis, thermal sclerostomy, trabeculotomy, goniotomy) or procedures to destroy the fluid-forming ciliary epithelial cells (cyclodiathermy, cycloelectrolysis, cyclocryopexy), direct surgery on the drainage canal of Schlemm. This also permits more detailed reconstruction of injured eyes and birth defects.

The mechanics of repairing retinal detachments have been so

refined that the likelihood of visual recovery has leaped from 50 percent to 95 percent in recent years, accompanied by a reduction in hospital stay from about six weeks to one week. Complex and difficult large detachments are now yielding. Extensive scarring, however, or strandlike formations in the vitreous or on the retinal surface present further mechanical problems in removal. Such excisions, vitrectomies, are currently done in most large eye centers under the "open-sky technique" in which the entire cornea is hinged backward from the glove, and surgery is conducted directly through the exposed vitreous face or by smaller incisions through the sclera and pars plana. At least for periods of several years, the vitreous body itself is now yielding successfully to careful surgical intervention and excision. Thus patients previously blinded with blood clots and fibrotic strand formation within the vitreous have been given new hope.

When dense clouding of the entire cornea makes it impossible to obtain a suitable nutrient host bed, it is now possible to consider the use of a clear plastic implant (keratoprosthesis) evolved by Hernandez Cordona, Columbia Presbyterian Institute of Ophthalmology. This is sometimes called the "nut and bolt" prosthesis which is anchored by screwing into the opaque cornea. Over 400 of these have been implanted. Although a significant percentage have been rejected by the tissue, a large number have remained in service for eight to ten years.

The Bronson-Turner metamagnet introduced about five years ago increases the magnetic flux (gauss) from a few hundred in the best of early magnets to approximately 10,000 gauss with this instrument. Operational usefulness at such high magnetic flux is limited to about 150 seconds due to concurrently generated heat, but this much time gives ample opportunity for critical extraction after localization of a foreign body. This hand-held magnet eliminates the encumbrance of the older "giant magnets" which were mounted on heavy coaster bases or high stands. New, low temperature research in "super-conductivity" poses the potential of even newer "super-magnets" which may increase the gauss yield by another log unit.

Progressive fractionation of treatment and use of lesser dosage of irradiation now can bring ocular and orbital cancers under control with markedly reduced x-ray damage to the sensitive eye. Immune therapy and lymphocyte transfusions offer effective promise of augmenting nature's defenses. Earlier use of radical surgical excisions has also increased the expectancy of cure and prolonged the outlook for sight and life.

At the moment, laser therapy offers the best possible way to obliterate new vascular tufts and seal vascular leaks. Its final role is not yet defined and the procedure is basically a destructive one. Generally, destructive forms of therapy are superceded as soon as secure knowledge of disease mechanism is achieved.

The advent of hydrophilic or "soft" contact lenses has been a mixed therapeutic and mercantile boon. Soft lenses can be used at least for a period of a few years to reduce hydrated corneas and fluid-filled epithelial blisters. They also may serve as repositories for drugs such as pilocarpine and some antibiotics. Durability is less than the well-known hard contact lenses made of acrylic or commercial products such as Plexiglas® and Lucite® plastics. All contact lenses still cause concurrent oxygen deprivation to the cornea, but the smaller corneal lenses have reduced this blocking.

Prognostic Advances

Careful and more numerous prospective studies of the natural course of ocular disease have given new prediction reliability to ophthalmologists. Similarly improved data concerning the eye's response to drugs and the interactions of multiple drugs have clarified principles of single and compound drug use. Therapeutic efficiency has distinctly increased. The more than 2,000 diseases now known to have genetically determined components also carry a large number of ocular involvements. This greatly facilitates prognosis within a family or sibship and for the offspring of known affected family members. The reliability of genetic counseling has increased greatly in the past few years and subsequently has come the improved biochemical therapy of a lesser number of genetically determined metabolic or enzymatic diseases. Genetic engineering or induced manipulation of the genes themselves is still some years away. The role of genetic advice is highly important among the blind and visually handicapped population, particularly because of the individuals' tendency to group around institutions designed for them.

Research Advances

The early years of electronmicroscopy offered a big jump in magnification beyond the usual upper limits of about 900× in light microscopy. Instrumental advances have now gone from the level of 200,000× to about 5,000,000×. A whole new world of minute systems within the individual cell is now visible to the human eyes of the researcher through high quality photographs at such magnifications. The total eye under such magnification would be larger than Mount Everest. Scanning electronmicroscopy also now gives a uniquely clear understanding of surface characteristics of the ultra-structural level.

The fundamentals of biochemistry are a common thread of physiology, pharmacology, bacteriology, and immunology as cells are explored. The details of intracellular organelles and the minuta of their functions are revealed chemically. Enzymes deficiencies are yielding to chemical replacement in a handful of disorders. Urinary screening for homocystinuria as well as phenylketonuria can identify and lead to correction of both serious ocular and mental disease.

The recent emergence of *clinical pharmacology* as a broadened discipline has linked the bedside therapist and the drug research laboratory in a productive intimacy not previously known. As the pharmacologist has come into greater symbiosis with the biochemist he takes new effectiveness to the planning of therapy. The highly complex organic formulae of modern antibiotics and drugs are much more thoroughly understood than in previous years, but their high effectivity is accompanied by some increase in side effects and adverse reaction.

Similarly the newly certified specialty of "nuclear medicine," a combination of pathology, radiology, and endocrinology, brings new specifics of radioimmune diagnosis and radioisotope therapy to the aid of many patients with neoplastic problems.

Cancer immunology, an exciting tool developed only during the last few years, is leading the way to the containment and neutralization of cancerous growths. It already has identified the reasons some tumors remain localized and others spread rapidly throughout the body. The potential for developing whole new strains of antitumor cells is real and near. Both the identification of tumor producing viruses and inhibiting agents, such as interferon and antimetabolites, offer vigorous though sometimes hazardous guns against cancer.

Both enzymatic alteration of aging in short life span animals (as the mosquitoes studied by Calvin Lang) and intracellular identification of components contributing to aging offer new specificity in maintaining cellular health. This in turn offers real potential for increasing bodily usefulness and life. Subtle factors in nutrition including trace metals such as zinc have been identified as vital to prolonged health. Positive fruits of aging research are reflected in part by recent increases in our advanced-age population. Septogenarians have increased by well over 100 percent since World War II and those over sixty-five have nearly doubled. These changes, however, call for increasing commitments to social and cultural planning for this burgeoning population segment.

References

Keeney, A. H.: *Ocular Examination: Basis and Techniques*, 2nd ed. St. Louis, Mosby, 1976, p.322.

Ruiz, R. S. and Avery, M. L.: *Ophthalmology for the Non-Ophthalmologist.* New York, Symposia Specialists, 1976, p. 80.

Martin-Doyle, J. L. C. and Kemp, M. H.: *A Synopsis of Ophthalmology.* John Wright and Sons, 1975, p.284.

CHAPTER 4

RECENT GENETIC ADVANCES IN THE DETECTION, PREVENTION, AND TREATMENT OF VISUAL HANDICAPS

HAROLD E. CROSS

GENETIC defects are a major cause of blindness and other forms of visual morbidity. More importantly, heritable ocular disorders in recent years are comprising an increasing proportion of blinding diseases. The reasons for this are at least two-fold. First, during the last two decades we have made significant progress in the medical and surgical therapy of many disabling nongenetic ocular conditions thereby reducing their proportionate contribution to the pool of visually disabling disorders. Second, and at least equally important, the virtual explosion in understanding and recognition of genetic factors in the causation of ocular abnormalities has made their role more obvious than was previously appreciated. In fact, it is doubtful that a book such as this even ten years ago would have included a chapter by a genetical ophthalmologist.

While it is true that most heritable disorders are individually rare, in the aggregate they are responsible for a significant proportion of eye disease, especially among younger individuals. Although accurate data are difficult to obtain, estimates from several studies are in remarkably close agreement. According to information collected by the National Society for the Prevention of Blindness, about 5.6 percent of all blindness in the United States in 1962 had an heredity basis.[1] Among blind children under seven years of age in 1965, genetic factors were cited as the most frequent cause, being reported in 47.4 percent of individuals.[2] Fraser and Friedman examined 776 blind children in England and Wales under twenty years of age (approximately 25 percent of the total number living in

28

England in 1963) and estimated that genetic defects were directly responsible for the visual handicap in 50 percent of cases.[3] These figures moreover must be considered minimum estimates since (a) rare disorders are frequently unrecognized and (b) the total number of heritable disorders is growing at an approximate rate of 10 percent compounded annually as new ones continually are being discovered.

Genetic diseases sometimes are considered rare forms of chronic diseases having little more than curiosity value with virtually no prospect for successful therapy. This view is no longer tenable in the light of recent advances in the detection, treatment, and prevention of genetic diseases. We now can look forward to a time in the not too distant future when a significant proportion of genetically determined visual handicaps will be eliminated or at least successfully treated.

The terminology and mechanics of heredity often are confusing to the nongeneticist; it is therefore essential to define several basic terms before outlining the major genetic mechanisms. The terms *congenital* and *heredity* often are incorrectly substituted for each other. Defects or abnormalities present at birth are, of course, *congenital,* whereas only those resulting from an error in the genetic material, i.e. in the genes, are truly *hereditary.* Congenital conditions include not only genetic disorders manifest at birth but also those that are due to birth trauma, intrauterine infections (e.g. rubella and toxoplasmosis), drug effects (e.g. thalidomide), and irradiation. Most abnormalities in the genetic information (genotypes) are present at conception, but since we usually recognize heritable disorders by their clinical manifestations (phenotypes), we do not consider the "disease" to be present until clinically evident, which may not be until adulthood.

The complete blueprint and instructions for each individual's unique development is encoded in the genes, half of which come from our paternal parent and the other half from the maternal mate. These genes consist of huge molecules of deoxyribonucleic acid, DNA, which serves as templates from which the appropriate enzymes and protein building blocks are synthesized. This process of *translation* takes place through a complex series of metabolic interactions and enzymatic steps which are incompletely understood in spite of remarkable advances in molecular biology in recent years.

Our genetic system also includes an almost foolproof mechanism for the duplication of genes to ensure faithful propagation of the species. Occasionally, however, changes in the DNA, known as *mutations*, do occur and if these are not corrected, clinical diseases often result. Since the change in DNA usually is permanent and hence transmitted to subsequent generations, we refer to these as heritable or genetic disorders.

Inherited abnormalities can be grouped into three major categories: (1) single gene mutations, (2) chromosomal aberrations, and (3) multigenic or multifactorial abnormalities. To understand recent contributions of medical genetics to the diagnosis, prevention, and treatment of visual handicaps, it is important to understand first the characteristics of diseases belonging to each of these groups.

Single gene mutations (sometimes called point mutations) usually produce characteristic clinical manifestations and therefore can be identified often as syndromes having a specific constellation of signs and symptoms. Examples of these among blinding disorders include classical retinitis pigmentosa, Best's macular dystrophy, Norrie's disease, and aniridia. The inheritance of such disorders is predictable since they are transmitted according to the laws of mendelian genetics. Point mutations occur in well-known patterns labeled by geneticists as autosomal recessive, autosomal dominant, sex-linked recessive, and sex-linked dominant.

Because the basic defect in single gene mutations involves a change in the molecular composition of the gene, its detection is beyond the limits of resolution of both light and electron microscopy. Fortunately, however, often the secondary biochemical change can be detected by appropriate laboratory tests. Like the specific molecular alteration in the gene, this metabolic change also is unique and thus provides a pathognomonic clue to the presence of the mutation. Improved techniques for the detection of these biochemical errors are among the most significant recent advances in the diagnosis of genetic disorders.

Chromosomal disorders result from the actual loss or addition of genetic material rather than an alteration in the molecular composition of single genes. Chromosomes are composed of giant linear arrays of multiple genes. Since recognition of chromosomal aberrations requires a relatively gross morphological alteration, large numbers of genes are usually involved. The clinical result therefore is far more detrimental to the individual than is a single gene mutation. In fact, the effect often is lethal with the result that the majority of affected conceptuses are aborted in the first trimester of gestation. Those that are carried to term usually have severe mental and physical defects. Two examples of chromosomal aberrations with significant ocular manifestations are Down's Syndrome (with cataracts and keratoconus) resulting from an extra number 21 chromosome, and trisomy 13-15 or Patau's syndrome in which retinal dysplasia frequently is present. Although occasional familial cases of chromosomal abnormalities are reported, most are not inherited in a predictable manner.

Not all heritable ocular diseases can be traced to single gene or chromosomal mutations. Many ocular characteristics result from the interaction of multiple factors, both genetic and environmental. These usually are designated as *multifactorial* in etiology. Since multiple genes often are involved, they also may be considered as multigenic conditions. Multifactorial disorders exhibit a wide range of clinical manifestations due to the variable nature and quantity of the causative factors. Multifactorial characteristics usually follow a "bell-shaped distribution" in degree of severity among the population depending upon the number of genes present and the particular environmental exposure of each individual. Such disorders, while frequently familial, do not occur in a predictable or recognizable pattern. Strabismus and refractive errors are examples of multifactorial conditions.

Aids To Genetic Diagnosis

Because environmental effects may produce diseases clinically indistinguishable from heritable disorders, the correct diagnosis is of vital importance before prevention or treatment can be considered. The significance of this is illustrated by a twenty-three-year-old, recently married female with optic atrophy who was referred to me for genetic counseling. She and her two sibs, one of whom also was affected, were the offspring of healthy, nonconsanguineous parents. Their condition had been diagnosed previously as hereditary optic atrophy at various medical centers throughout the country. Although the presence of optic atrophy in these patients was indisputable, there was simply no evidence that it was inherited despite the presence of two similar cases in a single family. The question of heredity was vitally important for the patient since she was anxious to start her own family. One clinical clue, namely, lack of any evidence of progression during the past twenty years, aroused my suspicions for this is uncharacteristic of known forms of hereditary optic atrophy. Further investigation revealed that both individuals during childhood received massive doses of antibiotics including chloramphenicol which is widely known to produce irreversible optic nerve damage in some cases. We are reasonably confident therefore that the risk of a similar problem among this patient's children is negligible since it was most likely caused by an environmental factor. On the other hand, ascribing the optic atrophy to a genetic mutation would mean that the risk of recurrence might be as high as 50 percent for each child.

Since biochemical anomalies are pathognomonic for single gene mutations, genetic diagnosis may be highly accurate provided the appropriate techniques are available. Advances in electrophoretic and chromatographic techniques have grown rapidly in recent years with the result that today there are at least seventy-five heritable metabolic disorders which can be detected in affected individuals (Table 4-I). In addition, the carrier heterozygotes, i.e. those who carry the mutation but are clinically normal, can be diagnosed similarly in sixty-three disorders (Table 4-II). Undoubtedly these lists will grow rapidly in the near future.

TABLE 4-I

GENETIC DISORDERS IN WHICH SPECIFIC METABOLIC
DEFECTS HAVE BEEN IDENTIFIED

Total: 75

Primarily systemic disorders with ocular manifestations: 9
    Albinism (Hermansky syndrome)   Tay-Sachs disease
    Alkaptonuria   Homocystinuria
    Fabry's disease   Nieman-Pick disease
    Galactosemia   Sulfite oxidase deficiency

Primarily ocular manifestations: 1
    Galactokinase deficiency

TABLE 4-II

GENETIC DISORDERS IN WHICH HETEROZYGOTES
CAN BE DETECTED BY BIOCHEMICAL ASSAY

Total: 63

Primarily systemic disorders with ocular manifestations: 6
    Cystinosis   Hurler's syndrome
    Galactosemia   Fabrys' disease
    Tay-Sachs disease   Hunter's syndrome

Primarily ocular manifestations: 1
    Galactokinase deficiency

As a practical matter, of course, it is possible to utilize such methods only if the biochemical defect is manifest in an accessible tissue or body fluid. Many genetic disorders, particularly those involving a single organ such as the eye, apparently do not manifestly alter the metabolism of other tissues and cannot be detected with current techniques. This accounts in part for the relatively few ocular disorders included in Tables 4-I and 4-II.

Chromosomal anomalies are detected through direct examination of the chromosomes. Since 1956, when suitable techniques for study of human chromosomes became available, the correlation of chromosomal abnormalities with certain complex disorders such as mongolism has made rapid progress. Until recently, however, it was not possible to identify each of the forty-six human chromosomes nor could small chromosomal segments be precisely localized to individual chromosome arms. However, newer fluorescent staining techniques developed in the past several years have removed these limitations with the result that cytogenetics now stands on the threshold of an exciting new era in genetic diagnosis.

Chromosome preparations are usually made from cells of the peripheral blood although it is possible to use those from any dividing tissue provided they can be cultured *in vitro* to obtain sufficient numbers for analysis. An inherent residual limitation in the study of chromosomal disorders is the inability to detect submicroscopic molecular alterations in the DNA. Fortunately, a number of human disorders involve either a change in the number of chromosomes or such gross structural rearrangement that detection is possible even with the light microscope.

Certain heritable ocular abnormalities such as Leber's congenital amaurosis and congenital glaucoma may already have caused permanent damage at birth. Obviously, any attempt to prevent or to treat such disorders will require prenatal detection. The recent application of amniocentesis techniques to the diagnosis of genetic disorders has made it possible to detect selected diseases as early as the first trimester of gestation. As shown in Table 4-III, at least twenty-five metabolic disorders, including seven with significant ocular manifestations, may now be diagnosed in this manner, with new ones being added constantly. In addition, chromosomal aberrations also can be detected in this manner.

Some heritable disorders may be diagnosed by direct analysis of either amniotic fluid or cells, whereas others require a more

TABLE 4-III

GENETIC DISORDERS IN WHICH PRENATAL DETECTION
IS OR MIGHT BE POSSIBLE*

Total: 25

Disorders with important ocular manifestations: 7
    Cystinosis   Homocystinuria
    Galactosemia†   Hurler's syndrome†
    Gaucher's disease   Hunter's syndrome
    Tay-Sachs disease†

*Not including chromosomal disorders
†Detected in utero

indirect approach. Examples of the former include Down's Syndrome in which chromosomes from the amniotic cells can be examined directly and Tay-Sachs disease where a deficiency in the enzyme hexosaminidase A can be detected in the fluid. Where such specific detection is not possible, one sometimes can take advantage of the sex-limited distribution of selected disorders. For example, ocular albinism, a sex-linked recessive condition which usually affects only males, cannot be detected *in utero.* However, female carriers of the gene can have normal children by carrying to term only female offspring, the sex of which may be determined by chromosome studies on the amniotic cells from each pregnancy.

Another indirect technique takes advantage of the linear association of specific genes located on a single chromosome since they generally are transmitted as a group to the next generation. This phenomenon, known as *linkage,* has as yet received only limited application in prenatal studies. The rationale is relatively simple — since genes located near each other on the same chromosome are inherited together with a known frequency, it is possible to estimate the probability that a given undetectable mutation is present provided another mutation located nearby can be detected *in utero.* Currently, only one such marker, the secretor gene, is located sufficiently close to another mutant gene, that of myotonic dystrophy, to be useful for such prediction.

Treatment and Prevention

At the present time and probably during the foreseeable future, specific therapy is available for only a few selected genetic disorders. One approach is through dietary modification such as in the case of phenylketonuria, galactosemia, and galactokinase deficiency. Another method which holds some promise is the supplementation of a missing factor to correct a metabolic deficiency. In at least two diseases with significant ocular manifestations, namely abetalipoproteinemia (Bassen-Kornzweig disease) and diffuse angiokeratoma (Fabry's disease), administration of both vitamin A and normal serum containing ceramide trihexosidase may provide at least a temporary amelioration of the clinical manifestations. A similar approach has had mixed success among the mucopolysacchariodoses. These systemic disorders of mucopolysacchariodoses metabolism commonly are manifest by clouding of the cornela stroma. Five or six basic types with a similar number of variations or subtypes can be identified by phenotypes or enzyme alterations. However, these methods in general provide only temporary relief and, of course, do not correct the genetic mutation. Optimistic reports in lay publications notwithstanding, it will likely be some time before actual substitution of mutant genes by "genetic surgery" will be practical.

This leaves us with the only other "therapeutic" alternative available at the moment — prevention of such disorders through genetic counseling and selection of normal conceptions. Changing attitudes toward the inevitability of such diseases together with more liberalized abortion laws now make it possible for most couples to exercise some choice in the selection of healthy offspring. This approach is not the ultimate answer, of course, since we would prefer to have methods by which we may select "mutationfree" germ cells for fertilization.

In this manner, we might be able to avoid the psychological and physical trauma that may accompany therapeutic abortions.

Accurate risk data are necessary prerequisites to making an intelligent decision by parents whose offspring carry a significant risk of inheriting a genetic disease. Armed with correct diagnosis, a complete family history, and knowledge of the mode of inheritance for a specific disease, it is possible to calculate the risk of occurrence among offspring. Actual risks vary from 100 percent to virtually zero depending on the specific disorder and the parental genetic background. However, the actual magnitude of the risk may be less important to the patient or family than the social and psychological factors which may influence the course of action taken by those who are seeking advice. For example, an emotionally well-adjusted and financially responsible childless couple may not allow a 25 percent risk of retinitis pigmentosa to dissuade them from having a child of their own, whereas a low income family with three or more affected children would be less likely to try again for a normal child in the face of similar odds. A genetic counselor should take these factors into account before presenting the actual risks, while realizing that the final decision will be made by those who seek the advice and not by the one who provides the data; strict objectivity must remain the cardinal rule for any counselor.

Summary

Heritable disorders constitute one of the major causes of blindness and visual handicaps, particularly among children and adolescents. Remarkable advances in diagnostic techniques have increased our awareness of their clinical significance although as yet relatively few can effectively be treated. The development of new approaches for treatment and prevention are desperately needed. In the meantime, earlier diagnosis *in utero* as well as genetic counseling can reduce substantially the morbidity until specific therapy becomes available.

References

1. National Society for the Prevention of Blindness: *Estimated Statistics on Blindness and Vision Problems.* New York, National Society for the Prevention of Blindness 1966.
2. Hatfield, E. M.: Blindness in infants and young children. *Sight-Saving Rev, 42:*69-89, 1972.
3. Fraser, G. R. and Friedmann, A. I.: *The Causes of Blindness in Children.* Baltimore, Johns Hopkins 1967.
4. Genetic Service: *International Directory,* 4th ed. White Plains, New York, The National Foundation 1973.

CHAPTER 5

THE OPHTHALMOLOGIST'S ROLE IN NEW REHABILITATION PATTERNS*

RICHARD E. HOOVER

ALTHOUGH the influence of several promi-
nent ophthalmologists on new rehabilitation patterns has been
sweeping, it has been largely unpublicized. It is the purpose of
this thesis to present information on their role in order to
enable other ophthalmologists to better equip themselves to
assist in the development of rehabilitation programs.

One of the most sought-after workers for the blind is "the
mobility instructor," a highly trained professional whose importance is substantiated by a current shortage. There is no
question that his competence and the philosophy which he
represents are two of the most useful and hopeful resources
brought to the service of blind people in our time. Again, it is
certain that he is the direct product of programs which could
not have begun or survived had not prominent ophthalmologists testified in the councils of government to the value of
these experimental programs. Mobility instructors now graduating from Boston College and Western Michigan University
were trained by instructors and resources developed at the
Veterans Hospital at Hines, Illinois. The program itself went
into operation against the advice of almost all officials, but
upon the insistence of Dr. James N. Greear,[10] then chief consultant in ophthalmology at the Veterans Administration Department of Medicine and Surgery. In both concept and personnel
it was the outgrowth of the United States Army Program at
Valley Forge, Dibble, and Avon, which had been founded
through the courageous insistence of Dr. Derrick T. Vail.[18] As

*From Richard E. Hoover, The Ophthalmologists's Role in New Rehabilitation
Patterns, *Journal of the American Ophthalmological Society*, *65*, 1967. Courtesy of the
Journal of the American Ophthalmological Society.

chief consultant in ophthalmology in the European Theater of Operations, Vail returned to the United States in 1944 to force through a dynamic, experimental program for blind soldiers, sailors, and veterans.

In exploring the usefulness of the "War Blind Group" of ophthalmologists, one must consider not only integrity and ability to command respect but also the methods which enabled them to enter this rather alien field successfully. Something, perhaps the large numbers of newly blinded people, caused them to reexamine what blindness actually means in basic terms of eating and drinking and even making love. This permitted them a view quite different from that of the "agencies" which were "accustomed" to blindness. Many of these agencies had grown more preoccupied with the problems of administration than of blindness. For better or worse, the army's problems of administration were well in hand; this brought the problem of blindness into high relief.

However appalled ophthalmological colonels may have been by the realities on their wards (including cane pounding and spilled milk), they faced them and set out to find solutions. As Gowman[9] and Greear[10] have shown the chief remedy was the sighted G.I. who "taught" the blinded person how to be blind. The agencies, who had originally been cool toward the War Blind Group, were now horrified. By 1946 the idea of the blind leader of the blind, which was so brilliantly exploited in the last century by Sir Francis Campbell, had become so nearly sacred that in adult programs at least it was almost a fundamental principle that all instructors of the blind be blind themselves. As alienation from formal work for the blind increased, so did the opportunity for experimentation. It was in such environments, unencumbered by old rituals, that new patterns began to develop. In fairness, it must be said that the army had in large numbers one element which the agencies had always lacked: personnel. However, it is also true that army personnel were willing to encourage the independence of blind people with true zeal for freeing them from custodial care. They saw plainly that this involved everyday practicalities.

People in work for the blind expected that ophthalmologists

charged with the War Blind Program in World War II would fail because the War Blind Program of World War I had been a failure. In the earlier program a revolution had been promised and none had ensued. It was whispered that ophthalmologists did not know how to handle the blind or what was best for them and that sooner or later ophthalmology would abandon the Blind Rehabilitation Program of World War II. The ophthalmologists made bad prophets of these skeptics. Two classic examples of this success were the World War II Army Program, the indisputable progenitor of the current peripatologists, and the Royal Normal College for the Blind, which would certainly not have come into being without the backing of Thomas Rodes Armitage, an ophthalmologist.

It has been a perplexing factor in the history of these important events in rehabilitation of the blind that the ophthalmologists who played such important influential roles have been so ready to vanish when their good deeds were done. Though it has undoubtedly been the mark of statecraft for them to allow others to take credit for their achievements, its negative aspect has been the continuance of a discouraging view of the ophthalmologist's role in rehabilitation which antedated World War II and which seems to have a tendency to spring up for obvious psychological reasons. Unfortunately this often deprives blind people of important influences which might benefit them.

The schools, workshops, and centers for the blind with which the public is familiar may lead to the erroneous belief that all blind people are collected in these places, where their problems and those of society are solved. However, the people at these centers represent only a small proportion of the blind population. The majority of the blind are scattered and integrated in the community: "Almost never is society put at a disadvantage because large numbers of blind people have suddenly appeared in a particular place."[1] This clarifies to some extent the diversified and often misinformed concepts found among many other ophthalmologists.

Simmons,[17] after interviews with several ophthalmologists, divided these members of the profession into three broad groups on the basis of their awareness and knowledge of the problems of the blind. Group one included those who had never sent a patient for rehabilitation services during their entire practice. One doctor revealed that when confronted with a severe problem involving marked visual loss, he sent the patient to the National Institutes of Health or Johns Hopkins for further diagnosis and therapy, and further, that if he should have a blind patient, he would send him to the Braille School in Baltimore, although there never had been one to send in twenty years of practice. (In fact, no such school exists.) His philosophy was, as he phrased it, "A sick eye resides in a sick body." And he maintained that these people have a very poor prognosis. In group two were those who leave no stone unturned, sending their patients to the National Institutes of Health and various institutions, but who are actually unfamiliar with agencies and their functions. The physicians in group three could cite cases of successful rehabilitation; they were aware of the severe problems a blind person must face and frequently had favorite agencies to which they referred their patients.

Before he became a physician, the author had an opportunity as an instructor of the blind to observe at first hand the early changes in this field. Subsequent experience as a physician and an ophthalmologist has engendered the hope that ophthalmology might be more helpful to blind people. In order to make the most humane use of his stature in the public mind and his access to blind people, the ophthalmologist should be familiar with certain basic information. All who enter this field wonder at first what is meant by talk of its multiplicity. In time they realize that blindness affects every aspect of human experience — the philosophy, theory, and technique of doing, thinking, and feeling, and always on an other-than-visual basis for performing.

The Physician

Exploratory studies reveal that 90 per cent of the blind seek medical care soon after the onset of serious eye symptoms. The eye physician, in addition to being one of the first professionals the blind person consults, symbolizes for the patient the ultimate in professional competence and knowledge in the area of visual impairment.

The ophthalmologist's role is fundamentally one of treatment, restoration, and prevention. Nevertheless, in the total medical program an understanding of medical therapy, surgery, safety, heredity, and rehabilitation are all necessary. Through training and experience the eye physician is competent in areas of health care, but may not always be prepared to envision rehabilitation as a part of medical therapy. The ophthalmologist's understanding of the area of visual impairment can be extremely beneficial to his patient. His potential power to encourage the use of rehabilitation services is great and his authority at a time of crisis may contribute significantly to future rehabilitative efforts. The patient senses his attitudes, expressed or unexpressed, and responds to them.

Information about condition and prognosis should be given as early as possible. The importance of this early timing must be emphasized. Hope for recovery or a miraculous cure when it is not justified is usually detrimental to the patient. The physician should not consciously or unconsciously feel guilty about the patient's visual condition or feel he has "let the patient down" if he cannot prevent loss of or restore vision. Yet such feelings may cause him to withhold a diagnosis of irreversibility and arouse a dangerous false hope.

The ophthalmologist should be able to envision rehabilitation as well as medical and surgical care. He need not equate poverty with the need for service or think only in terms of jobs or vocational training. His understanding should encompass training in social services, recreation, education, home care, child care, self care, communicative skills, mobility, and vocations. The lack of such knowledge is inevitably reflected in the care and counselling of the blind patient. The ophthalmologist need not be a psychologist or a psychiatrist, but he should be aware of the need for psychological security. Carroll[2] has designated as threats to this security losses affecting physical integrity, confidence in the remaining senses, reality contact with the environment, visual background, and light security.

The Blind

The most widely accepted definition of blindness in the United States had its inception in the deliberations of the House of Delegates of the American Medical Association in its 85th Annual Session held in Cleveland, Ohio, in June 1934. The definition states: "A person shall be considered blind whose central visual acuity does not exceed 20/200 in the better eye with correcting lenses or whose visual acuity, if better than 20/200, has a limit to the central field of vision to such a degree that its widest diameter subtends an angle of no greater than twenty degrees." Like all aging covenants, it must be respected till the world can negotiate a better formula.[12] It has become firmly entrenched in the lives and thoughts of physicians and the public. Yet, an honest analysis of the definition reveals its inadequacies as a means of identifying with any degree of preciseness those who are visually disabled, since it leaves the physician without guidelines to predict and direct rehabilitative services. To determine statutory blindness, only two visual characteristics need to be measured. These are the best corrected visual acuity for distance or the central fields, if the visual acuity is better than 20/200. There is no requirement concerning standardization of lighting, test charts, or distances for visual acuity, and no mention of size, color, or distance of test objects in determining field capacity.

In other words since the definition specifies no levels of disability, it implies that all have the same visual impairments, or that all good doctors have such rapport that uniformity is automatic. Since this is not the case, the physician must assess disability as well as impairment, without prior standards of visual measurement to help determine visual ability or disability. It is comparatively easy to assess someone as totally blind and thus totally visually disabled. It is often difficult to evaluate visual ability or disability in the person who has less than total loss of the sense of vision.

Peckham says: "The potential ability of the partially sighted for peripheral response, either of rods or cones or both can provide a guide in attempting to assist the patient with visual aids. Subjective estimation of the remaining visual capability is quite difficult to obtain: The patient cannot explain why he cannot see. . . . Our usual habit of depending upon macular vision and of assessing all visual response by macular response is fallacious."[15] He recommends objective tests to assess the retinal response of the rods, cones, and ganglion cells differentially.

The customary definition embodies two dictionary definitions — the blind who have no sense of vision, and the cecutients who are visually impaired. The blind are also either masculine or feminine. They are either congenitally or adventitiously blinded. If they have been adventitiously blinded, it could have occurred at any age after birth and existed for any length of time. They can be of any age and any intelligence, and have additional handicaps, other medical problems, and a wide diversity of training, aptitude, interests, and experience.

An increase in blindness is predicted.[13] Even if it were not, it is such an important world health problem that interested physicians should understand the rehabilitative as well as the medical and surgical care of these people. In this regard, they should realize that there is a "how" they see and a "what" they see, since only about one-quarter of the estimated 500,000 "blind" are totally so. The practical and psychological problems associated with "blindness" are significant and intimately affect medical and rehabilitative care.

The Problems of the Blind

The totally blind (those without useful light perception) are much easier to categorize than the cecutients (those with partial sight) and so in most ways are easier to mold into a rehabilitative pattern. The cecutient is faced with a myriad of visual problems, as well as the social, psychological, and financial problems and basic skill losses he holds in common with the totally blind person.

In view of the tendency to play down one's own inadequacies

and disabilities, whatever they may be, it is surprising how little sympathetic understanding people extend to those with severe sensory deprivation (such as severe visual loss) who may not wish to be labeled "handicapped" or "blind." Although their protests are not always eloquent, many are so sensitive that they might go hungry rather than accept the gratuities for the blind.[8] In certain areas the habit of applying the word "blind" to those who have useful vision persists. Physicians and service workers alike have an obligation to respect the feelings of those who see poorly, but who do see. They are not without the sense of vision and usually do not want to be considered sightless, which denies the blessing of whatever sight they have. Blindness is the ultimate of visual loss which the person with sight fears with a special intensity.

When his blindness occurs the permanently blind person loses his ability to manage in the world by visual means. It is a devastating impairment; but the sooner he is informed, and understands, recognizes, and accepts this total irreversible loss, the sooner he will become efficient in his management of a dark world. The cecutient, however, loses his ability to manage by visual means many times during the day, month, or year. Nevertheless, on occasion and under certain conditions he uses vision. People who retain even a small remnant of the sense of vision use it for certain tasks no matter how inefficient or painful it becomes.

It is a rehabilitation maxim that one can only be rehabilitated at the level of the impairment. Failure to consider those with severe but not total visual loss in the aid of the "blind" has had subtle effects on medicine, program planning, and services. It is a partial denial of the basic principle that people are individual in their problems and needs. A visually impaired person cannot be rehabilitated as totally blind. All processes must unite to incorporate the remaining vision into as effective and efficient a system of personal management as possible. The dynamics of emotional adjustment are very similar in all cases, however, differing primarily in intensity, duration, and stability of adjustment.

It is important to recognize that the cecutient has a built-in ambiguity: he must be brought to realize that it will be difficult for the public, friends, associates, and professionals to fully understand his needs for special aids and techniques in certain areas and situations when in other areas and at other times he apparently functions as a normally sighted person. There is a body of ophthalmological knowledge which can help these people identify areas and situations in which special aids and techniques are necessary. Such a person must become skilled in interpreting his impairment to others when situations demand it.

There are three avenues open for the cecutient, but only one offers a reasonably serene and full life. If the cecutient withdraws into a familiar and unchanging environment which can be well controlled with his visual capacity, he restricts his potential unnecessarily. If he continues to live the full life, enduring the hardships, inconveniences, dangers, and misunderstandings which are an integral part of his life, he is labeled at times "a charlatan," "a fake," "a malingerer," even "a drunk." The emotional and physical drain often causes him to operate physiologically on a razor's edge. It adversely affects his sense of well-being, creates great anxiety, and can jeopardize both his personal safety and that of others. The only truly effective course is for the person to maintain an objective viewpoint toward the restrictions and assets his vision affords him and to reorganize his attitudes, skills, techniques, and aids. The informed physician and trained rehabilitation personnel should direct therapy to this end. The patient's success depends on the practicability of the overall reorganization. It is not an easy task and takes his maximum efforts as well as continued professional interpretation of the nature and extent of his impairment.

The totally blind person unquestionably has losses which not even the cecutient faces to the same degree. His disability is psychologically more shattering because of its finality and threat of lifelong duration. There are a myriad of repeated frustrations in the daily life of the totally blind which reemphasize the helplessness and dependence of the condition. It is "soup with a fork" thousands of times during the working day.

Eating, alone, can cause so many problems, embarrassments, and frustrations it is a wonder more blind people do not give up the effort to eat normally and revert to the bib and fingers. As Carroll says,[2] "try it yourself sometime — the blindfold dinner technique. It won't teach you about blindness, but it will teach your about this phase of blindness." Acts of personal hygiene, dressing, shaving, grooming, shopping, telephoning, running a house, keeping accounts, putting away the groceries, sorting the mail, lighting a cigarette, finding the ash tray or the waste paper basket, cleaning the desk or the room are just a few of the problems which force dependence and the embarrassment it engenders.

Of the twenty losses described by Carroll[2] there are two which are particularly significant in the practical scheme of everyday living. They are the loss of mobility and orientation skills, and the loss of communicative skills as ordinarily performed with a normal sense of vision. Unless one can continue to move from place to place and to read and write, one's world becomes woefully constricted and restrictive. These losses are of different degree, intensity, and direction, but they do occur and constitute major losses for both the cecutient and the blind. The ophthalmologist is in a key position to direct and encourage therapy beyond the usual concept of diagnosis, medicine, and surgery.

Communicative Skills

A variety of solutions to the problems of blindness have been available for some time and new ones are always being proposed and requested. It takes precious development time to put scientific principles to work in routinely usable instruments. Consequently, by the time responsible investigators are ready to try a few reliable prototypes in the field, technology has advanced to a point where the prospective users know or dream of something smaller, lighter, more informative, and cheaper. Frequently, the product is felt to be obsolete even before a good analysis of its worth is attempted. Known ways of circumventing the loss of vision rely heavily on the use of auditory or tactile senses, but one cannot interfere with the other and one cannot present information in a less efficient way than is practical and pleasant.*

In spite of this mass of technical knowledge, there are still many potential devices which would be simple and useful to the blind in their everyday lives but which are not yet available. Frequently requested are methods and devices for the following purposes:

to make pie dough of uniform thickness;

to cook pancakes, eggs, and various types of meats in a frying pan;

to indicate when the typing is within three or four lines of the bottom of a page;

for a blind typist to make erasures and corrections;

for a blind person, living in a rural environment, to find the gate to his yard when returning home, or to locate the gate so he can shovel a path in the snow from his front door to this gate in the winter time;

to center a piece of material for turning on a lathe;

to make duplicate turnings on a lathe;

to solder materials, such as wires in electrical equipment;

for reading the volume control on the microphone when recording material on tape;

to indicate when a blind person is reaching the end of a spool of tape when recording on it;

to join narrow boards together and thus make a wide board for a table top, shelf, or similar project;

to enable a blind craftsman to sharpen his own chisels, hand or planer blades;

to enable a blind person to cut materials in wood or metal, using a pattern as a guide;

to read a level manually and by ear.

Students and blind persons in professions want a braille

---

*For the most up to date international listing of educational, household, personal, recreational, vocational, and medical devices including thermometers, insulin syringes, hygrometers, and optical probes, the reader is referred to *Proceedings of International Congress on Technology and Blindness*, Volume 4, Catalogue Appendix. New York, The American Foundation for the Blind, 1963.

stylus that will not cause as much muscle fatigue as the present instrument when they have to write braille for several hours at a time under conditions where it is impractical to use the braille writer. Blind persons operating precision equipment in factories need micrometers, calipers, and various types of gauges that will enable them to measure materials at very close tolerances. Such tools should be suitable for a blind person of average ability, not just the exceptional individual.

There is enough familiarity with the typewriter, the talking book, the tape recorder, large type print, and braille that depth discussion here would not be meaningful. At the same time, the great need to provide the blind with a far greater wealth of literature than can ever be made available by any of the above methods must be emphasized. A device to translate the written or printed word and present it to the blind in the form of auditory or tactual information in a pleasantly acceptable manner and at a practical rate of speed would be exceedingly worthwhile and useful. The idea has been under study at various times during the past fifty years. It received new impetus during and after World War II and the Veterans Administration deserves credit for keeping interest and research active in this area.

There are two broad approaches being intensely explored. One is a direct coding machine which converts printed text scanned by a photoelectric sensing device into sound patterns bearing some relationship to the letter shapes. The reader has to learn to recognize the sounds and associate them with the printed letters. So far, machines of this type have been cumbersome, unreliable, and tedious and have not gained common acceptance. The other type of machine widely considered differs from the first one in that the machine itself is responsible for recognition at the letter level and could possibly produce spelled speech sounds or connected speech at the output. It is quite apparent that a machine producing ordinary speech is the best solution, but at the moment technical and economic difficulties make it unlikely to be available for personal or private ownership for many years to come.[16] Until then, the time-honored and well-tested reading and writing methods of braille, talking books, tape recorders, and the typewriter must suffice for those whose visual ability is insufficient to resolve the written and printed word.

Orientation and Mobility

For those who are deprived of the visual ability to maintain control of physical position and movement from place to place, the loss of orientation and mobility is probably the greatest. Historically, the stick, staff, or cane has been the most common tool to help overcome this loss.[11] However, certain animals have contributed their skill and services as guides, and from the beginning of time the seeing people have, of course, acted as guides for those who could not see.

The author intends to develop this subject rather thoroughly since developments in a hospital setting during World War II were directly responsible for the advances since 1960 in the graduate training of mobility and orientation instructors (peripathologists) to propagate techniques and aids in travel. These new ideas and training methods at first met great resistance but have now proven to be one of the greatest contributions to new rehabilitation programming.

Experience at Valley Forge General Hospital during World War II where a large number of people with severe eye injuries were grouped for eye care and rehabilitation purposes emphasized the need for expert ophthalmological guidance in all skill areas. Probably the earliest of all help for the blind in this realm is the human helper, companion, or guide. Even today, the human guide has an important role in the orientation and mobility life of the blind, whether he is the physician in the office, the nurse or aide in the hospital, the parent or kin in the home, or the friend or stranger on the street and in the bus, plane, or cab. Yet few people know the principles and philosophy of guiding, directing, or moving with the blind. This became such a monumental problem in a hospital setting that a basic set of principles and techniques were developed by Hoover, Bledsoe, and Tigani[14] for use by those who would be with the blind.

A uniform method of protection was adopted to eliminate the natural inadequate attempts at groping to which so many people without sight resort. Either the right or the left arm can be used: the upper arm is held at right angles to the shoulder and parallel to the floor, while the forearm is held parallel to the floor at right angles to the upper arm with fingers extended and relaxed to protect the far side of the body. For even the most awkward this method gives adequate protection against door jambs, posts, and half-opened doors which might damage the face or eyes.

No one should assume that he knows more about the patient than the patient himself does. It must always be remembered that the blind person did not lose his wits when he lost his sight. If he is treated as though he had, it will be reflected in this loss of respect for the doctor and for himself. People have a tendency to shout at those who cannot see. This, of course, is unnecessary. On the other hand, one must not mumble; since the patient depends on his hearing, one should speak distinctly. One knows that he is not doing this if the patient keeps asking one to repeat what was said.

The individual's medical condition should be the physician's primary concern. No matter how well qualified in this area, he should not talk on unexplored subjects. Compensation benefits, state benefits, methods of learning braille, and typing may or may not be foreign, but there are people who know about these things and know how to explain their usefulness. One should especially avoid careless talk about "the wonderful things science is doing." A newly blinded individual may need help in certain areas, but one should remember to give only as much help as is necessary.

It is discourteous to speak to the patient through his kin or through a friend, unless the patient is a child and does not understand the implications of what is being said.

Strangers will often speak to the patient through the doctor if the opportunity arises. If this occurs, the physician should always refer the question to the blind person; this usually can be done very diplomatically.

If the patient is to be guided, the proper procedure is for the guide to ask the patient to take his arm. If it is necessary to make some slight movement to get out of the way or maneuver into position, to sit down or get up, he must direct the patient in doing it. This is not done by shoving or by propelling. One does not take his hand and move it from him unless it is necessary to show him some particular object, at which time the action is prefaced by saying "Let me show you."

In directing a patient or person who is blind to do something in the hospital or office, one should be particularly careful to picture carefully what move the patient is about to make in order that exact directions may be given. Special care should be taken to avoid mixing right and left. This is frequently done when one is facing a person and can cause much confusion. If a patient has been guided to a place and left alone, one should be sure that he understands his location. It is usually better, under such circumstances, to establish some point of contact, such as a counter, chair, table, or wall.

Rarely is anything done well in confusion, particularly in the case of people without sight. This should be kept in mind and pains should be taken at all times to avoid mix-ups, indecision, and upheavals in plans.

The patient or client is as capable of observing the rules of courteous behaviour as he always has been, even though he cannot see. He will expect to shake hands on being introduced but since he will not see an offered hand, it must be presented to him in a way which is comfortable and convenient for him to locate. It should always be made clear when one is leaving a person who cannot see; one should never leave the person talking when he is not there; and he should always tell the patient when he comes back.

The expressions "over there," and "right there" should be used sparingly. Instead, one uses "Let me show you," to fill up the time lag until one can establish contact between the patient and the object or chair to which he is directed.

One must be careful in offering examples of what other blind persons can do. An individual must learn about this in a natural way from general conversation. One never knows to what level an individual may rise; therefore, it is unwise to underline the achievements of others in such a way that he feels inferior.

Articles should not disappear from a patient's reach as if by magic. If it is necessary to move his personal belongings, or some object which he uses regularly, he must be told it is being moved and where.

If entering a confined space such as a small examining cubicle, an examining chair, or an automobile, a person can engineer his own actions better if one hand is placed on something like the door handle or some other familiar object and the other in an area where he might accidentally bump his head. Then the situation will be familiar enough to suggest the whole picture to him. If he becomes confused, further information can be given, but no more than one person should take over in such cases. In public places or in noisy places where there is confusion, a person will need much more help than in quiet, familiar surroundings. Many of the things he ordinarily does with ease in his own environment will become difficult in a different place.

Many well-meaning people try to help the person who is blind but do not know how. Frequent questions of people without sight are, "Where will I be able to find you?" "How will I get hold of you?" and "Will you be there?" It is very unpleasant for a patient who cannot see to be kept waiting, since he cannot scout for himself when there is a delay. One should always be definite in making appointments, be prompt in meeting him, and give the patient an alternative course of action in case of an emergency which might prevent one from meeting him.

As one observes patients in the hospital setting who have both eyes patched after surgery, are totally blind, or have serious eye trouble so that they cannot see, one notices that eating becomes a great challenge. The nurse or aide should always tell the patient when she delivers the tray to the bed and when she removes it. The tray should be removed as soon as possible after the patient has finished eating. When the tray is brought the patient should be told what is on his tray and where it is. This should be done slowly enough that the patient has time to visualize what is there.

For a new patient food should be served bite size and whatever is not cut in this manner should be so cut by the person who delivers the tray. The plate should be turned so that starchy foods form a wall for slippery foods. Usually this means keeping the starchy food at the left or at the back of the plate. For new patients, bread should be buttered, and, as desired, sugar should be placed in the beverages. Cereals from boxes should be placed in a bowl and sugar and cream put on them; food should be salted and peppered as desired. Although a patient is to receive the service just described, a person who does not regain vision eventually will have to learn to serve himself. Eating skillfully by touch consists mainly in doings things just as seeing people do, but taking pains and paying far more strict attention. Certain tricks common among people without sight may be shown to the patient, although in the main he will develop his own. Suggestions in regard to doing more complicated things for himself may be given to a patient by people who are experts — not while he is eating, but in casual conversation between meals followed by a practical demonstration later. In sugaring food, the patient will find it helpful to let his hand travel ahead toward the dish about to be sugared. This will not only give direction, but the height of the cup or dish toward which he is aiming.

Cutting meat is the most difficult operation for the blind person to perform at the table. Most people who are well-informed on the subject agree that it is not an undue surrender of independence for this service to be done by someone else, especially if the knife is dull and the meal is to be enjoyed. Food may be salted and peppered by dusting salt and pepper through the fingers extended over the dish. Other people prefer to pour the salt into the palm and scatter it. To avoid the use of fingers, a piece of bread may be used as a backstop in the left hand while the food is taken up onto the fork.

It is usually impossible for a blind person to have a reliable human guide at his beck and call and the only other travel aids in common use are the dog guide or cane. In the west the earliest written evidence of the use of dogs as guides is an account by Trevisa in *The Olde English Translation* (1398) from the comments of a monk named Bartholomew on contemporary life about 1260: "The unfortunate conditions of a blind man are so great, that it makes him not only subject to being led by a child or by a servant but also by a dog."[4] The modern story of dogs as guides for the blind originated with Dorothy Harrison Eustis, who bred and trained dogs for specialized duties in the Swiss army and who in 1927 wrote an article for the *Saturday Evening Post* telling of her observations on the use and training of shepherd dogs in Germany to lead blinded German veterans of World War I. Mrs. Eustis trained the first dog to be used by a blind American. Her article entitled "The Seeing Eye" so caught the fancy of the public that most people refer to all dogs guiding blind people as seeing eye dogs.[4]

There are about a dozen guide schools in the United States, but the largest and best of its kind in the world is The Seeing Eye, Inc. at Morristown, New Jersey. Only its trained dogs can be correctly termed Seeing Eye™ dogs. The Seeing Eye, Inc. is in its thirty-eighth year and has placed approximately 3100 trained dogs with blind travelers. Even if all schools were of equal duration and caliber, it is apparent that there is still need for travel aids and techniques to accommodate the many thousands newly blinded each year. In 1960 the Research Center of the New York School of Social Work[6] prepared a study called, "The Demand for Dog Guides and Travel Adjustment of Blind Persons." This study points out the desire of most blind people to improve their travel performance and the lack of active plans on the part of most to accomplish this. It further demonstrates a surplus of facilities for dog guide programs, while cane programs are in insufficient supply to meet existing needs.

The use of electronic, ultrasonic, and mechanical equipment as guiding devices for the blind appeals to the motorized and mechanized public so that considerable effort and publicity has gone into the research and possible development of such aids, either as supplements to or replacements for the human, dog, or cane as travel guides and aids. The original research began as a result of early experiments by the author and Colonel Gordon Chambers in the use of an interrupted light source which directed its beam at an object. The reflection of the light source was captured and transformed into audible signals which by proper coding could measure (within certain limits) the distance of an object from the traveler. This idea was transferred to the Signal Corps of the United States Army and under the supervision and direction of Cranberg[5] and his colleagues, the first prototypes of this device were produced and field tested. At about this same time, in January of 1944, the Committee on Sensory Devices of the National Research Council, under the chairmanship of George W. Corner, had its first meeting. This committee arranged contracts with the Brush Development Company, the Hoover Company, the Stromberg-Carlson Company, and the Franklin Institute of Philadelphia, each of which developed portable instruments of sufficient power to permit ranging for later testing at Haskins Laboratories.[20] From this simple beginning has stemmed a large and complex research and development program.

In general there are two types of devices being studied: energy radiating devices, which must be very thrifty in their expenditure of energy, and passive or ambient devices which require less energy but have high false alarm rates. Current devices are experimental and must be recognized as environmental sensors or object detectors which might become especially useful as supplements to the cane or dog guide.*

The proper cane used correctly can be the most valuable aid yet available to the majority of the "blind." One must remember it is only an aid, and that to travel competently from place to place, the blind cane user must not only be familiar with the cane touch technique but must be able to listen and use what he hears. Most blind travelers say that hearing is the most valuable orientation sense. Underdevelopment or lack of such clues either from ignorance, pathology, or unawareness prevents top-quality orientation to one's surroundings. The

---

*For the most complete international listing of special purpose and adaptive mobility devices, the reader is referred to *Proceedings of the International Congress on Technology and Blindness*, Volume 4. Catalogue Appendix, New York. The American Foundation for the Blind, 1963, and the *Proceedings of the Rotterdam Mobility Research Conference*, The American Foundation for the Blind, May 1965.

tactile sense transmitted primarily through the fingers, hands, and feet and through the cane to the fingers and hand is also a valuable orientation and travel tool. It must also be isolated, developed, and taught. It is obvious the olfactory sense can also be useful. Many establishments such as bakeries, markets, barber shops, flower stands, and candy and peanut shops can give valuable orientation clues to the blind travelers. Proper training techniques can also improve the use of this sense.

Even if all senses are exceedingly acute and superbly trained, the blind traveler still needs to know first whether there is a safe platform on which to step and whether there are objects in the path which would lead to injury or embarrassment if undetected and unnegotiated. This is just what the correct cane properly used can tell him.

In trying to teach techniques in the use of the cane as a travel aid to hundreds of the newly blinded it was soon discovered that the customary white cane was inadequate. Similarly, individual systems developed by some blind travelers could not be universally adopted. An attack on these two problems was made by the author and his staff. The design and characteristics of the perfect cane were analyzed. First of all, it should be just long enough to inform the user of a safe spot on which to place his next step, a length that will differ with each traveler. It must be light in weight so as not to cause fatigue. There should be a grip, crook, or handle which allows ease of handling and perfect control without finger cramps, palm sweating, or annoyance from extreme temperatures. There should be a durable tip which does not wear too rapidly or stick too badly when being touched to terrain, but which dampens none of the desirable tactile and audible information it should be reporting. The shaft itself should be durable and properly conductive — transmitting tactile and audible clues but avoiding undesirable or dangerous conductions such as electricity, cold, heat, and unnecessary noise. It would be convenient if it were telescopic or easily collapsible to allow for easy storage when not in use — as in trains, buses, planes, restaurants, and china shops. If possible it should be attractive. The color is individual and not necessarily white. The white cane, such a popular image of the blind in this country, was adopted as a national promotion project by the International Lions Club Convention in Toronto in 1931. As a result local ordinances and state laws have been passed concerning their use and significance. But blind persons who wish instead to use canes of other hues are at liberty to do so, and their own skill and judgment in managing the cane can be much more dependable than the dubious advantage of being spotted by a motorist on a modern highway. The cane is currently regarded as a symbol of independence and not one of dependence. Its value now lies in its proper use and not in its specific color.

After more than twenty years of interest and probably less than fifty dollars in direct research there is not yet the utopian cane. However, through the interest of the Somerill Tubing Company's executives and engineers at Norristown, Pennsylvania, canes were designed, built, and supplied in numbers to the eye service at the Valley Forge General Hospital. The canes met most of the necessary specifications; however, modifications and innovations of this original design have been numerous.

The problem of finding a technique that made the best use of a good cane remained. The user needed to determine the presence of a safe platform on which to step, to avoid all dangerous and embarrassing objects from the waist down, and to determine steps down and steps up. The cane makes no claims to find objects hanging from above, to maintain balance and direction, to plan directions, or to otherwise fulfill the requirements of muscle, nerve, hearing, smell, or touch other than that immediately conveyed as the cane touches the terrain with each step taken. It can be used as a bumper in certain areas and under certain conditions and there are designated techniques for this specialized use. Its real value is in negotiating ever-changing and unfamiliar environments.

When the cane is used in an uncontrolled environment the hand gripping the cane is dropped in a natural position to the side. The dorsal aspect of the elbow is then rotated inward slightly so that it rests firmly on the hip bone, and the hand holding the cane moves to a comfortable, moderately relaxed position in the very center of the body slightly below waist level and very close. The cane is held at the proximal end with the weight supported comfortably against the thenar eminence and guided largely by the thumb and index finger. With the forearm remaining stationary the hand moves back and forth pointing the cane so that the tip describes an arc before the user. This arc should never rise more than one or two inches above the ground and should always touch the spot where the advancing or rear foot is about to be placed, thus ensuring that there is no obstruction but solid safety for the advancing foot.

If a traffic intersection is to be negotiated the orientation and techniques are very specific and involved and will not be detailed here. However, since ascending or descending steps is often a hair-raising experience even for the normally sighted, the somewhat condensed description of technique is included to show the logic and safety involved.

When the tip of the cane indicates the presence of a drop or a step down, the first thing which must be ascertained is the depth of a step. This should be done by putting the cane down on the second step and moving forward until both toes extend over the edge of the step the same distance when the heels are parallel. In this way good direction is obtained. If there is a succession of steps, the next important thing is the width of the tread, which is found by moving the tip of the cane forward until the edge of the second step is located. Then, it is important to know if there is a margin of safety on either side in order that one may not step off the side in case there is no wall or banister. This is done in one sweeping motion of the tip of the cane along the edge of the second step from about twelve inches past the left side of the body to approximately twelve inches past the right side of the body. Now the traveler is ready to descend, with the hand holding the cane falling naturally at the side and the tip of the cane extending past the edge of the second step and two or three inches in front of it. The cane and hand are held motionless, the traveler tilts the head forward as if looking where he is going, for this gives better balance, and descends with a relaxed, normal gait. If the cane and hand have not been moved during the descent, the tip of the cane will touch when the bottom of the steps has been reached. The foot/cane rhythm is then resumed.[11]

This does not complete in detail all the intricacies of cane use, but it is specific enough to familiarize the physician with the mechanics and notion of the cane's design, characteristics, and effectiveness.

So important has this concept of orientation and mobility become that in 1960 the Vocational Rehabilitation Administration of the Department of Health, Education, and Welfare sponsored the first school of peripatology to be founded — in the School of Special Education at Boston College. This educational program and training leads to a master's degree in special education. Since then, departments have also been established at Western Michigan University and California State College at Los Angeles. Others are in prospect and interest in undergraduate training in this specialty is also beginning to prosper. This means that qualified instructors with master's degrees will soon be available in agencies, schools, centers, and hospitals to supervise, direct, and teach these important skills.

Ophthalmologic Influences

The literature is scant concerning the role of the ophthalmologist in relation to the social and emotional adjustment of his patients. Cholden[3] presented one of the few systematic treatments of this problem. The Research Center of the New York School of Social Work, Columbia University, attempted to determine by questionnaire if there was fairly consistent agreement among ophthalmologists on a core of rehabilitative concepts and principles. The profile of majority concepts listed below could be used as a set of standards for the ophthalmologist interested in rehabilitation care.[7]

1. A broad concept of the role of the ophthalmologist is held, one going beyond specifically medical concerns. Positive attention to the long-range social and psychological adjustment of blind persons is held to be an opththalmologist's concern.

2. The ophthalmologist has awareness and concern for such problems accompanying blindness as economic need, impaired travel ability, psychological difficulties in adjusting to blindness, and difficulties in relating to people.

3. Information to patients as to the condition of blindness should be given early, so that rehabilitative measures may be begun as soon as possible. The manner of informing patients should keep individual characteristics and situations in mind.

4. Hope for recovery should not be left when the condition of blindness is clear and irreversible, as it will interfere with readjustment and rehabilitation.

5. The ophthalmolgist has the major responsibility for informing the patient of his condition, though he may also enlist the aid of others.

6. Expectations for the social role of blind patients should be similar to those for sighted persons, with optimism as to the possibility for reasonably happy and useful living. Specifically, economic self-support, emotional independence, and satisfactions in work and in relations with others are held to constitute elements of the satisfactory adjustment of blind persons, just as they do for sighted persons.

7. Active referral of patients for social rehabilitation services of various kinds, including travel training, is favored. Guidance, referral, and continued interest in the adjustment of blind patients are considered to be important accompaniments of practice in informing patients of blindness.

Cultural stereotypes of the blind man either make him out a beggar, a complete dependent, social and economic inferior, or portray him as a blind genius who can tell colors, has facial vision, can do "the most extraordinary and wonderful things," and has unusual hearing, tactile, and perceptive abilities which the seeing do not have. Unfortunately, the first stereotype is the most prominent so that sighted people feel that life and social position as a blind man may be untenable.

The doctor may feel blindness to be a loss of his own self-esteem and prestige or a damaging reflection to his professional reputation. It is certainly important that the ophthalmologist's attitude toward blindness should be clear; otherwise, it will further confuse the already devastating picture blindness has for the patient. It is difficult to tell a person he is irrevocably blind. It is easier to insinuate or hold out a hope that the person may some day see again through a medical or surgical miracle. Hope for recovery, so important therapeutically in most aspects of medicine, is a cruelty to the permanently blind and a major deterrent to his adjustment.

The physician is by training and service a humanitarian, and his motivation in holding out a hope of seeing is quite humanitarian. He does not want to be cruel at any time, and especially in the intimate confines of the hospital room or office, he finds it cruel to condemn anyone to a blind person's life of dependency. At the same time, he is in a key position to inspire the blind person to improve or rebuild his life. This he must do with knowledge, courage, conviction, and simplicity. The patient can sense a doctor's attitudes and convictions. With the secure knowledge that there are ways, means, devices, and activities with which the blind can continue to be socially and economically productive and emotionally stable, he need not view a blind man's lot as one of uselessness.

Conclusion

In conclusion, it should be reemphasized that the ophthalmologist can have an important role in developing new concepts for the rehabilitative care of the visually impaired.

The departure from traditional approaches to rehabilitation therapy for the blind as experienced and performed in a hospital center in the 1940s met with opposition, especially as it related to the need for improvement in communicative and mobility skills.

With support from a few ophthalmologists and the use of new techniques and aids centered around orientation and mobility, the blind section at the Veterans Administration Hospital, Hines, Illinois, operates as the living proof of the merits of this new concept and of the value of this new therapy.[19] Its current dynamic importance is reflected in plans by the Veterans Administration to open other centers of a similar kind. It is further demonstrated by the organization of graduate schools of orientation and mobility at Boston College, Western Michigan University, and California State College at Los Angeles and by the persistent demand for graduates of these programs as instructors in schools, communities, agencies, hospitals, workshops, and rehabilitation centers.

References

1. Bledsoe, C. E. and Williams, R. C.: The vision needed to nurse the blind. *Am J Nursing, 66:*71, 1966.
2. Carroll, T. J.: *Blindness.* Boston, Little, 1961.
3. Cholden, L. S.: *A Psychiatrist Works with Blindness.* New York, Am Foun Blind, 1958.
4. Coon, N.: *A Brief History of Dog Guides for the Blind.* New Jersey, The Seeing Eye, 1959.
5. Cranberg, L: Sensory aid for the blind. *Electronics, 19:*116, 1946.
6. Finestone, S., Lukoff, I., and Whiteman, M.: *The Demand for Guide Dogs and the Travel Adjustment of Blind Persons.* New York, Columbia University, 1960.
7. Finestone, S. and Gold, S.: *The Role of the Ophthalmologist in the Rehabilitation of Blind Patients.* New York, Am Foun Blind, 1959.
8. Froestad, W. M.: The partially seeing aren't blind. *New Outlook for the Blind, 60:*239, 1966.
9. Gowman, A. C.: *The War Blind in the American Social Structure.* New York, Am Foun Blind, 1957.
10. Greear, J. N.: Rehabilitation of the blinded soldier. *New Outlook for the Blind, 40:*271, 1946.
11. Hoover, R. E.: The cane as a travel aid. In Zahl, P. A. (Ed.): *Blindness.* New York, Hafner, 1962.
12. Hoover, R. E.: Toward a new definition of blindness. In American Association of Workers for the Blind: *Blindness.* Washington, D. C., AAWB, 1964.
13. Hoover, R. E.: Vision — the most valuable sense. *Wilson Lib Bull, 40:*818, 1966.
14. Hoover, R. E., Bledsoe, E. W., and Tigani, W.: *Guide for Those Giving Rehabilitation Services to the Blind.* Intraservice publication for the

Office of the Surgeon General, 1945.

15. Peckham, R. H.: *The Visual Responses of the Partially Sighted.* HEW, Vocational Rehabilitation Administration, Contract No. RD 1382-S. Washington, D. C., U. S. Govt Print Office.

16. Nye, P. W.: Reading aids for blind people — a survey of progress with the technological and human problems. *Med Electron Biol Engng, 12*:247, 1964.

17. Simmons, R. E.: Ophthalmological attitudes toward rehabilitation of patients with loss of vision. *New Outlook for the Blind, 60*:299, 1966.

18. Vail, E. T.: The veterans administration program for the training of the blinded serviceman. *Am J Ophth, 35*:1457, 1951.

19. Williams, R. C.: Therapy for the newly blinded as practiced with veterans. *JAMA, 158*:811, 1955.

20. Zahl, P. A. (Ed.): *Blindness.* New York, Hafner, 1962.

CHAPTER 6

DIABETICS: A NEW GROWING AND SPECIAL CONTINGENT OF CASES

Frank L. Myers

IT is a distinct pleasure for me to participate in the development of this book because I sincerely believe it is a book that is long overdue. The main reason my chapter, the diabetic patient, is in the book is illustrated in Figure 6-1. In 1970, diabetic retinopathy ranked second as a cause of new blindness in the model reporting area for blindness statistics and was the leading cause of blindness in the forty-one to sixty year age group.[1] It should be noted that blindness was defined as a visual acuity of 20/200 or less or visual field less than 20°. Thus, although senile macular degeneration was the leading cause of so-called legal blindness, we know that this condition rarely causes total blindness. In contrast, a large number of diabetic blind have substantial visual field loss, as well as central visual loss. It is not news to most ophthalmologists that diabetic retinopathy has become one of their major problems today. I doubt that this is news to the rest of you, but I think it is worthwhile emphasizing the point with a few additional statistics.[2] In 1970, there were 43.6 diabetics per 1000 general population. This is predicted to double by the year 2000. In 1970, it was estimated that there were 154,000 blind diabetics in this country. If the present rate of new blindness continues, it is predicted that there will be 573,000 blind diabetics by the year 2000. There are, as yet, no good solid statistics concerning the chances of an individual diabetic becoming blind. We must also keep in mind that the prognosis for life in blind diabetics is not good. The best current estimate for patients who have developed proliferative diabetic retinopathy is that 40 percent of patients are dead in five years and 50 percent of the survivors are blind.

FOUR LEADING CAUSES OF BLINDNESS

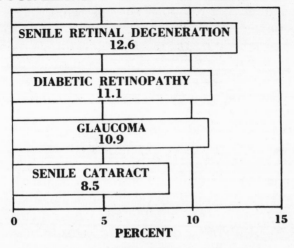

Figure 6-1.

What causes blindness in diabetics? In a study of our cases in 1968 (Table 6-I) four major reasons were identified: (1) severe vitreous hemorrhage, (2) retinal detachment, (3) macular edema, and (4) neovascular glaucoma.[3] The latter is usually a "final blow" to an eye that is already blind from one of the other causes and at the present time remains virtually incurable.

TABLE 6-I

CAUSES OF VISUAL LOSS IN DIABETES[3]
(200 EYES WITH 20/40 OR LESS FOR
SIX MONTHS OR MORE)

VITREOUS HEMORRHAGE	33 percent
DETACHMENT OR DISTORTION OF MACULA	30 percent
MACULAR EDEMA OR EXUDATE	22 percent
NEOVASCULAR GLAUCOMA	13 percent

It is obvious from looking at Table 6-I that diabetic

retinopathy is a complicated and multifaceted disease with many variations. For example, vitreous hemorrhages often are intermittent and in many clear spontaneously. The patient thus may have a variable degree of vision loss for a variable length of time. This makes it very difficult to predict the kind of visual problems an individual patient will have and when he should be referred for rehabilitation counseling, declared legally blind, etc.

In order to understand where the various causes of visual loss fit into the overall picture, I would like to review the natural history of diabetic retinopathy and then discuss briefly some current modes of treatment. Diabetic retinopathy initially becomes manifest as a few "red dots" in the retina. These are saccular outpouchings from the retinal capillaries and are called microaneurysms. They may be indistinguishable from small hemorrhages also within the substance of the retina. The wall of a microaneurysm may be thin and allow leakage of fluid from the blood into the retina, causing swelling or edema of the retina. Later deposition of fat molecules from the edema fluid forms yellowish-colored "hard exudates." These and several other ophthalmoscopically visible lesions make up what is called nonproliferative or "background" diabetic retinopathy (Figure 6-2). If edema of the retina from leaky microaneurysms involves the macula, then central visual loss will occur. The basic cause of these changes is not known, but we do know from pathologic studies that there is loss of the capillaries in the retina which results in decreased circulation and poor oxygenation of the retina. Capillary loss is a retinal manifestation of a more generalized involvement of the small blood vessels of the body organs in diabetics called microangiopathy. It has been postulated that microaneurysms are an abortive attempt at formation of new capillaries to replace those lost.

When actual new vessels not previously present are formed, an advanced stage of the disease called proliferative diabetic retinopathy begins. Proliferative diabetic retinopathy develops in a certain percentage of diabetics with background retinopathy. The proportion that go on to develop proliferative retinopathy is not known precisely but has been estimated to be as

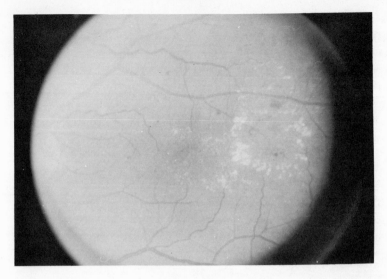

Figure 6-2.

high as one third. Newly formed vessels break through the inner membrane of the retina from the substance of the retina to grow on its surface. They may remain dormant for years but usually a process called vitreous contraction intervenes. Shrinkage of the vitreous is the basis for the vitreous hemorrhage and retinal detachment that are the major causes of visual loss in proliferative diabetic retinopathy. In this process, the vitreous gel contracts into a smaller volume than it previously occupied, pulling away from the retina. The newly formed vessels on the surface of the retina are adherent to the back surface (the posterior hyaloid face) of the vitreous and are pulled forward from the retinal surface. In the process, the thin walls of the vessels may be stretched and torn, and hemorrhage into the vitreous occurs. Later, the vessels may regress as fibrous tissue accompanying them proliferates and a scar tissue adhesion between the shrunken vitreous and the retina is formed (Figure 6-3). If further contraction of the vitreous occurs, traction is exerted on the retina and the retina is pulled forward, resulting in retinal detachment. If this involves the central retina and macula, visual acuity is markedly affected. Even if retinal detachment does not develop and vitreous hemorrhage in time clears, profound visual loss can result from marked sclerosis of the retinal circulation. However, retention of a surprising degree of visual function oftentimes occurs in the "burned out" phase of retinopathy. When this stage is finally reached, progression of the various lesions stops and whatever visual function is left remains stable or deteriorates slowly from gradual degenerative changes of the macula or from cataract formation.

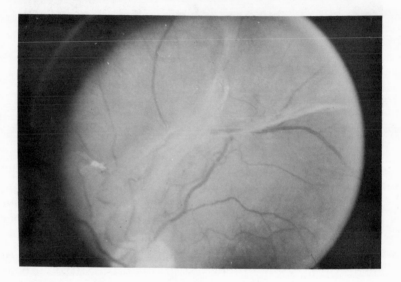

Figure 6-3.

As noted previously, neovascular glaucoma may intervene at any stage and cause loss of function in an eye. In this process, newly formed vessels grow on the surface of the iris occluding the channels of outflow of the aqueous humor from the eye. Elevated intraocular pressure, congestion, and pain in the eye develops. While pain and congestion can be treated medically, control of the increased pressure is very difficult and usually unsuccessful.

The treatment of diabetic retinopathy at the present time remains difficult and the results are hard to predict. This is largely a reflection of the variability of the disease. Efforts at the present time are directed toward (1) elimination of macular edema, (2) prevention of vitreous hemorrhage, (3) removal of vitreous hemorrhage, and (4) repair of retinal detachment. Although, in the past, various operative procedures to destroy the anterior pituitary gland were used because there was some evidence this prevented progression of neovascularization, the serious nature of the procedure and potential complications have led to a decreasing number of these operations being done. Instead, photocoagulation treatment is being used in most centers today. This treatment utilizes an intense beam of light which, when focused on the retina, burns and shrinks the abnormal new vessels. The light may be white light generated by a powerful xenon arc light bulb or a green light generated by an argon laser. A nationwide cooperative study involving sixteen centers throughout the country (the Diabetic Retinopathy Study or DRS) is currently underway to try to determine the effectiveness of this treatment. In this study, only one eye of a patient is treated because of possible harmful effects on the eye by the treatment itself. Considerable destruction and loss of visual field may occur from the treatment, and it is not known if the treatment may stimulate contraction of the vitreous or the formation of fibrous scar tissue.

Recently, preliminary results of this study have been reported and indicate that in certain selected types of proliferative retinopathy photocoagulation is beneficial in reducing severe visual loss at least over a two-year period.[4] The study is an ongoing one, and further results and possibly additional types of proliferative retinopathy that might be benefitted by photocoagulation treatment are anticipated.

In addition, an exciting new operation called vitrectomy has recently been developed to remove old hemorrhage clouding the vitreous jelly. An instrument is inserted into the center of the eye through a small incision (Figure 6-4), and small amounts of opaque vitreous are nibbled up and removed while being replaced by clear fluid. Our recent experience with this operation in diabetic vitreous hemorrhage has shown that 60 to 70 percent of cases can be improved.[5]

Some of the most difficult cases needing treatment are those

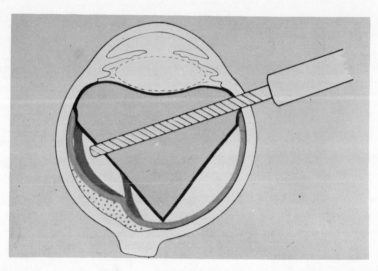

Figure 6-4.

with diabetic retinal detachments. Many of these eyes cannot be helped by surgery. Scleral buckling operations can be successful when a retinal tear is present and closed; but in many instances, the detachment involves vitreous traction on the retina with considerable scar tissue formation. Vitrectomy may offer hope for some of these cases in the future but there will remain cases in which visual function cannot be restored.

In summary, I would like to suggest that the diabetic patient presents one of the most challenging problems to the medical and allied professions. These patients have a crying need for comprehensive and coordinated care. In addition to the need for multiple specialty treatment, they have impressive social problems which are too often ignored as we concentrate on the medical dysfunctions. Rehabilitation is difficult because of the multitude of problems; and, unfortunately, there is a tendency among some of us to feel that they are not worth our time because of the poor prognosis for life. This is especially true when it comes to the older diabetic.

Furthermore, the newly blinded diabetic has considerable psychological problems that are not well comprehended by many rehabilitation personnel who are blind but have been so since birth. There is a tendency for these individuals to have unexpressed resentments which, if verbalized, would go something like this: "Well, you're not so bad off. At least you had vision for a considerable period of your life. Look what I've done and I never had vision!" Psychologically, however, the person who has had good vision and then suddenly loses it has considerably more problems than one who has never experienced good vision. This whole problem is akin to the depression encountered by quadraplegics and is well recognized by rehabilitation personnel in these areas. Considerable work needs to be done in the analogous situation in the newly blinded.

These people need support, guidance, and specific help and recommendations instead of admonitions to "quit feeling sorry for yourself and get to work." Because of their neurologic, cardiac, and renal problems, they often are unable to be totally rehabilitated; but, at least, we should extend ourselves to help them make the most of what abilities they do have. These tragic individuals are no less deserving of our best efforts. The rewards that come from attempting to meet their challenge can indeed be gratifying.

References

1. Kahn, H. A. and Moorhead, H. B.: *Statistics on Blindness in the Model Reporting Area, 1969-1970.* HEW, Publication No. (NIH) 73-427. Washington, D. C., U. S. Govt Print Office, 1973.
2. Kanarek, P.: Diabetic retinopathy and blindness: Estimates of decennial prevalence rates. Harvard School of Public Health, unpublished data prepared for Richard Field, The Retina Foundation, Boston, 1970.
3. Myers, F. L., Davis, M. D., and Magli, Y. L.: The national course of diabetic retinopathy: A clinical study of 321 eyes followed one year or more. In Goldberg, M. and Fine, S. L. (Eds): *Symposium on The Treatment of Diabetic Retinopathy.* Public Health Service, Publication No. 1890. Washington, D. C., U. S. Govt Print Office, 1969.
4. The Diabetic Retinopathy Study Research Group: Preliminary report on effects of photocoagulation therapy. *Am J Ophthalmol, 81*:383, 1976.
5. Myers, F. L. and Bresnick, G. H. Vitrectomy in diabetic retinopathy. *Trans Am Acad Ophthalmol Otolaryngol,81*:OP-399, 1976.

CHAPTER 7

LOW VISION AIDS PROGRAMS

BENJAMIN MILDER

THE Visual Aid Clinic in the Department of Ophthalmology at the Washington University School of Medicine has been in existence since 1958, and while it may differ in some respects from other such programs, it is representative of university-affiliated low vision projects. There are some 120 centers in existence, not all of which are functioning effectively. Despite the small number of such facilities, it is likely that most of you have some degree of familiarity with the existing programs and with the types of functions which they perform.

There are more than four million partially sighted persons in this country, with about 10 percent being added to the total each year. Even if all centers were performing at maximum efficiency and capability, there would still be only one such center for every 35,000 visually handicapped individuals. Thus, there is an appalling inadequacy of visual aid services. Those centers which exist are significantly maldistributed with the concentration being in big cities and the teaching centers in medicine and optometry. On the brighter side, however, the American Foundation For the Blind has been charged with, and is undertaking, an in-depth study of the distribution of these services, with the goal of improving the availability of such centers. To this end, a full-time project director has been employed and an advisory committee is already at work.

At Washington University, St. Louis, Missouri, the Visual Aids Clinic is a subspecialty division of the Department of Ophthalmology and originally was funded by the Office of Vocational Rehabilitation of the Department of Health, Education, and Welfare as a demonstration project, from 1958 until 1962, for the stated purpose of evaluating the role of visual aids

74

in rehabilitation. The clinic, now maintained by the Department of Ophthalmology, has the following goals: (1) community service, specifically providing vocational and social rehabilitative services, (2) a teaching resource in the training of ophthalmology residents, and (3) a research function. Patients are seen by referral from the university ophthalmology clinic, from private physicians, and from government and private service agencies. The study of each patient includes an evaluation of his referral data, a medical and social history, an ophthalmologic examination (where this does not accompany the patient), refraction examination for glasses, and testing with specific visual aids. An appropriate aid (or aids) is then selected for the patient and wherever possible the visual aid device is loaned to the patient for a trial at home or under his work conditions. If the trial is successful, the visual aid is prescribed and the patient is seen subsequently to evaluate his performance.

An examination for a visual aid is not qualitatively different from the examination of any eye patient but does differ in several specifics. First, the patient's history and his *specific* visual requirements are of critical interest since the visual requirements may be quite circumscribed, in comparison to those of the normally sighted person. Second, the examination techniques must be pursued deliberately and slowly because the patient with limited vision cannot respond as rapidly or as accurately as his normally sighted peer. Finally, these patients require a maximum of support and reinforcement during examination procedures and during follow-up care.

By general consensus, the term "partially sighted" has been used to describe those patients whose vision is not correctable beyond 20/70, but a better definition of "partially sighted" would be "anyone unable to achieve his visual goals and needs with conventional spectacle lenses." By this latter definition, there are many perfectly happy, well-adjusted individuals who can see no better than, for example, 20/100 and who neither desire nor require any form of optical aid. These are the patients who are sometimes mistakenly labeled as "lacking motivation" when in reality what they lack is "need." Optical aids, by definition, are "devices intended to maximize the available vision in any partially sighted person," including the so-called "legally blind."

The Patient Profile

Who is the person cared for at the Visual Aids Clinic? There is no stereotype. Patients have been seen ranging from age five to age ninety. Success in benefiting from a visual aid is, in general, related to the amount of available vision. It is obvious that a person who can see 20/100 is more likely to be fitted successfully and to use successfully a visual aid than the person who has only 4/200 vision. Success also is related to the degree to which the patient can modify his acuity by accommodation. By utilizing maximum accommodation, a short focal length can be achieved, with resulting increased magnification. Thus a child with 20/200 distance vision may read well using a weak optical aid or even none.

Success in the use of an aid does not depend, for the most part, upon the nature of the disease process which has caused the visual impairment, but there are exceptions. Specifically, those diseases which are accompanied by a marked reduction of the peripheral field of vision generally yield poor candidates for help with a visual device. Patients with advanced glaucoma and retinitis pigmentosa are illustrative of this group. On the other hand, youngsters with poor vision resulting from congenital nystagmus and albinism seem to do quite well with visual aids and success rates here approximate 100 percent. For all other diagnostic categories, between 60 and 70 percent of the patients could be fitted successfully with some form of optical aid.

Once it has been determined that the patient is capable of seeing adequately with a visual device, his success in adapting to that device will depend upon such factors as his intelligence, his educational background, a realistic appraisal of his needs, and his specific visual goals. To a large degree it will depend upon his motivation.

Working with the partially sighted patient is a source of considerable gratification to the physician or optometrist because of the high proportion of patients who can be benefited. At the Washington University clinics, two thirds of all of the patients could be fitted successfully with some visual aid device. Of those patients whose visual acuity was 20/200 in the better eye with conventional spectacle lenses, 70 percent could be made to read twelve point type. Even with vision as low as 5/200, 20 percent of these patients could be fitted with an optical device which enabled them to read eight point type!

How Optical Aids Work

Most frequently, the vision problem of the partially sighted individual resolves itself down to an inability of the central part of the retina (the macular area) to receive sharp images, while the peripheral retina is relatively less affected. By enlarging the image on the retina sufficiently to spread it over an area larger than the affected central portion, the patient may be made to see satisfactorily. Thus, our goal is to achieve *magnification* of the retinal image. This can be performed in a number of ways.

1. If the patient moves closer to the object of regard, the image on the retina becomes larger. If the patient who is having difficulty seeing his television set at nine feet pulls his chair up to three feet away, his linear image becomes three times as large and the television screen becomes nine times as large. By the same token, if one holds reading material closer to the eye, the print is magnified. Unfortunately, as one moves through the adult years, the accommodation decreases, so that when we hold objects close enough to magnify in that fashion, the images are too blurred to be interpreted correctly. However, small children, who have maximum capability of adjusting the focus for near, are able to read for prolonged periods of time while holding the printed page at such short distances as two or three inches from the eyes. (When printed matter, normally held twelve to thirteen inches away, is moved to three inches, linear magnification is increased four times.)

2. When we use lenses to magnify the image, what the lens

actually is doing is improving the focusing capability of the eye and shortening the focal distance so that the magnified image will be seen clearly at very short distances. Thus, it is the *short distance* from the eye which provides the magnification, and the lens enables the eye to see clearly at that short distance.

3. Telescopes function in a different manner optically and provide a larger image on the retina without moving the image plane closer.

Successful use of an optical aid will depend on the degree of sensory depression at the macula or area of central vision in the retina, i.e. visual acuity, but will depend to a greater extent on the breadth, or *area* of the retina, involved.

Optical Aids

Optical Aids for Distance Vision

About one of every five patients at the Washington University clinic receives, in addition to a device to assist for reading and close tasks, some form of optical aid to assist his distance vision. The most common beneficial device to improve distance vision is a properly prescribed pair of eyeglasses. It is not uncommon to find patients with markedly limited vision which can be improved substantially by the correct lenses.

When appropriately fitted lenses do not aid significantly in distance vision, one can resort to *telescopes*. These may be in the form of headborne telescopes worn much like spectacles for both eyes or the same type of telescope used as a monocular device. The conventional *prism binoculars* such as those used at sporting events provide an excellent form of telescopic device. Compact forms of prism binoculars or prism monoculars (to be used with one eye) are available. Clip-on monocular telescopes and compact prism monoculars were generally unknown fifteen years ago. Some telescopic lenses are small and may be fitted into or cemented onto ordinary spectacle-type carrying lenses. Finally, some patients with limited vision are benefited by *contact lenses*. Patients with keratoconus, who cannot benefit greatly from spectacle lenses, may achieve substantial visual improvement through the use of contact lenses.

Telescopic devices to aid distance vision have several pronounced drawbacks. The field of vision is quite small, there is a disturbing sensation of movement of the objects as the telescope is moved (motion parallax), and they are, at best, bulky. They function most satisfactorily in static situations — classrooms, meetings, theatre, and other situations where one cannot magnify the object by moving closer.

Optical Aids for Near Vision

Once again, one of the most frequently used and effective aids to near vision is a careful and accurate refraction examination and the prescribing of a proper pair of glasses. Beyond this, a large variety of "head-borne" magnifying devices is available.

Strong *converging (convex) lenses* in spectacle frames may provide needed magnification. The ability to produce these very strong lenses in so-called *aspheric* form reduces aberrations and provides a larger clear field of vision, and they are available in light-weight plastic. They, too, have been developed during the past fifteen years. These also may be prescribed as half glasses or bifocals, thereby allowing the patient to use the upper portion of his field of vision for orientation and mobility, and the lower part for reading tasks.

More recently, strong lenses of this sort have become available in the form of thin plastic sheets of varying power up to twenty diopters, using the principles of the *Fresnel* (or ship's lantern) lens. These sheets can be simply moistened and pressed on the existing glasses. They can be cut with a scissors and made to simulate a bifocal, or applied to the patient's existing glasses in any form. They provide an excellent temporary method of determining the effectiveness of magnification devices for a patient.

Telescopes, such those described previously for distance vision, can be combined with a reading cap and used for close work activities. Such a device offers the advantage that it enables one to hold the reading material at a greater distance than a spectacle lens of corresponding strength. This may be necessary for writing and for certain vocational activities.

Various forms of *loupes* are available for both binocular and monocular use. Small loupes, such as worn by jewelers, are readily clipped onto the patient's existing glasses.

The most commonly employed magnification devices are *hand-held magnifiers* and almost every partially sighted individual has obtained, on his own, one or more of these devices at the dimestore, drugstore, or from an optician. These magnify in the same manner as spectacle-type magnifiers. They have the advantage of a more comfortable working distance for short duration. Although they have a rather small field, they are useful for looking at prices, telephone directories, and catalogues, and they have the great advantage of being small and portable.

Stand magnifiers have the same characteristics as hand magnifiers except that they are placed on the reading material and a fixed distance between the lens and the reading material can be maintained. They may be a fixed focus type of stand magnifier such as a plastic aspheric "cataract reader," or they may be adjustable, such as with a Sloan focusable stand magnifier. In this latter lens, the distance from the lens to the paper can be adjusted slightly to take care of a moderate refractive error in the patient's eye. They may also be illuminated and illumination is indispensable when a relatively high-powered magnifying lens is needed. Paper-weight magnifiers, such as the Visolett®, provide uniform diffuse illumination over the reading field and are quite useful when a low-power magnifier is indicated.

The best, and most frequently required, nonoptical aid to impaired vision is *increased illumination.* When the magnifier requires a very small focusing distance, the patient's head causes shadows and illumination is essential. Compact, high intensity lamps can be brought to within a few inches of the visual task, when needed. In some cases, however, when the visual impairment is due to abnormalities of the ocular media

— scarred corneas, cataracts, and opacities in the vitreous humor — bright illumination is a deterrent to useful vision. *Line guides* are helpful in enabling the patient to maintain his orientation when reading and a *reading stand* is almost essential for the patient using a strong magnifying device. *Nylon point and brush point pens* and laundry markers are useful for increasing the legibility of the written word. Rulers, watches, and telephone dials are available with enlarged markings and numerals. *Large print* magazines and newspapers are available, although they are limited in scope. Patients most frequently can read ordinary newsprint equally well by the use of magnification devices, although the working distance may be compromised.

Closed circuit television devices, for magnification of print, have been developed within the past few years. These devices have been promoted vigorously by the manufacturers, and their poor acceptance by the visually handicapped is not to be interpreted as any failure on the part of the advertising media but rather due to their cost which is in the range of $1500 to $2500 each. In actual fact, these devices do not provide a substitute or improvement over the magnification devices described above. They do provide a very useful extension of these devices, however, because they are capable of achieving considerably greater magnification — up to forty times (equivalent to an improbable 60 diopter lens!).

The Role of the Visual Aids Clinic

The selection and prescription of an appropriate aid or aids represents only the beginning of visual rehabilitation. *Training* the patient in the use of the aids and their specific application to his vocational needs presents the larger problem confronting the rehabilitation forces. If it is true that an on-going effort is involved after our rather extensive study, what then is the particular advantage of a visual aid center? There are several. First, there is the ability to give the patient all of the *time* necessary to evaluate and resolve his visual problem. More time is required than the average physician would be able to devote to these problems even if he were sufficiently motivated. Second, into such a center can be brought a sufficient number of *devices* so that the most suitable can be tested and various aids can be *loaned* to the patient for home or job trial. Third, a *team effort* can be made available in the visual aid center, including in many instances the services of the ophthalmic or optometric technician, and the social worker as well as the ophthalmologist or optometrist. Finally, most of these patients have a history of disappointment and discouragement. The presence of such a specialized clinic improves the potential for the patient's acceptance of the corrective device. There is the attitude that they have come to the "court of last resort" and in these specialized surroundings some expertise is available which can be applied to their visual problems.

The real question is: what do we accomplish with all of these efforts, in a rehabilitative sense? Early in our original studies, we found that we had to define "rehabilitation." In the school-age population, any improvement in the information-getting capability was rehabilitative, in the sense of broadening the horizons for study and ultimately for work opportunities. In the older population, the ability to read one's own mail, sign a check, or find a telephone number was rehabilitative in the sense of reducing dependency upon another family member.

However, in the more restricted sense of rehabilitation as an economic goal, as a means of restoring a person to self-sufficiency, does the visual aid clinic materially improve the chances of achieving this result? Our visual aid clinic reviewed fifty consecutive patients referred by the Missouri Vocational Rehabilitation Division. Of these, thirty four were between the ages of twenty and sixty. Twenty-nine of these patients received some form of optical aid; fifteen of them reported good utilization of their optical aids, three reported fair utilization, and none were described as having poor utilization. Now the ability to use the optical aid does not necessarily mean that the patient was able to be rehabilitated so that he was able to make use of the aid in the job situation for which he was being trained. Of the twenty-nine patients, nine found their optical aid to be of some value in rehabilitation and twelve found them of no value in the particular job which they performed or aspired to perform. Thus, nine of the original fifty referred patients were what we would call "successes." Whether this is a good result or poor result becomes more of a matter of philosophy than of statistics. As I see it, aiding eighteen percent of a group of previously unemployable individuals is a dramatic success and it is apparent that increasing our training in the use of these aids would add to the success rate.

Over the years, the visual aid clinic has rehabilitated, in an economic sense, persons in the following activities:

artists	college students
mechanics	electronic workers
farmers	clergy
doctors	assembly line workers
typists	salesmen
musicians	bankers
school teachers	

What's New

I am reminded of our cataract surgical technique. It differs little from the operative procedure of three months ago and that was little different from the one used a year ago. However, if it is compared with the cataract operation I performed thirty years ago, the changes seem to be quite dramatic. So it is with optical and visual aids. Changes come slowly and gradually, but they come.

So, if your ask, "What is new in the field of visual care for the partially sighted?" I would mention the following:

1. *Teaching* — There is a broadening base of exposure to this field in ophthalmological residency programs and in schools of optometry.

2. *Paramedical Training* — Centers are now crystallizing programs for the training of ophthalmic and optometric technicians, as technician aides in the field of eye care. Some of these trainees will find their careers in a visual aid center.

3. *Technology* — Programs for wider dissemination of closed circuit television will increase the range of visually handi-

capped who can be rehabilitated. Lens devices will improve in sophistication.

4. *Field of Education* — Educators are becoming increasingly aware of the range of available aids and are decreasing their dependence on large print reading material. They have discovered that print size can be doubled as easily with a 2✗ magnifier as at the printing press.

5. *Nationally* — There is an awareness of the gross inadequacy of visual aid centers — in numbers, distribution, and services. Activities such as those of the American Foundation for the Blind are certain to yield great dividends for the partially-sighted of this country.

In summary, it is evident that visual aid centers are inadequate in numbers and that the delivery of visual aid services and devices is inadequate in the United States. The potential for economic rehabilitation of the partially-sighted person is significant, and economics are as attractive to the partially-sighted as to anyone else.

Bibliography

Faye, E. E.: *The Low Vision Patient.* New York, Grune, 1970.

Fonda, G.: *Management of the Patient with Subnormal Vision.* St. Louis, Mosby, 1970.

Keeney, A. H.: Field loss vs central magnification. *Arch Ophth, 92*:273, 1974.

Low vision services in the united states, *Sight-Sav Rev, 43*:223-226, 1973.

Milder, B.: Visual rehabilitation for the near blind, *Mo Med,* pp. 1353-1357, November 1960.

Sloan, L. L.: *Recommended Aids for the Partially Sighted.* New York, National Society for the Prevention of Blindness.

CHAPTER 8

VISUAL MEASUREMENTS AND FUNCTIONAL CLASSIFICATION IN RELATION TO ASSISTANCE DEVICES

LORRAINE H. MARCHI

"THE PLAGUE" for centuries of human history was a general name given to prevailing occurrences of illnesses carrying off great numbers of people. There is little known about the modes of communication of early plagues. They occurred where a large population was crowded together, especially in warm climates. The earliest recorded history of a plague was described by Thucydides as occurring in the second year of the Peloponnesian War in 430 BC.

General histories always include descriptions of two major plagues. The Justinian Plague, which took place in 544 AD in Constantinople, raged so violently that 1,000 gravediggers are said to have been insufficient for the interment of the dead. The greatest plague of all was the Black Death which ravaged the civilized world between 1348 and 1350. In Europe alone over twenty-five million died — between one quarter and one half of the total population.

We now understand, because of discoveries by such giants as Jenner and Pasteur, that plagues were several illnesses caused by different viruses. The progress of medical science has been, to some extent, the identification of these viruses and their classification so that research can address itself meaningfully to treatment approaches.

Through our Medical Advisory Board, the National Association for Visually Handicapped has established a one-page outline classifying the visually impaired into diagnostic groupings based upon the Snellen notations which are not easily translatable into working guides. These groupings bridge the needs between ophthalmologic notations and functional capabilities of the visually impaired. We believe this will aid the professional in meeting the needs of visually handicapped persons by the use of this simplified outline.

The diagnostic group has been divided into four main areas:

I. Blindness which includes three subgroupings: (A) no light perception, (B) light perception and projection, and (C) central acuity up to hand movements and with gross field loss. This category's functional guidelines include the use of braille, dog, cane, and/or a device wherein the lack of vision is not a deterrent, as well as stressing for the totally blind the use of optical to sensory conversion techniques.

II. Hand movements to 2/200 with restricted field — lists in the functional equivalent, marginal form vision and assistance of light localization.

III. Includes those with central acuity of 2/200 up to 10/200 with form field exceeding twenty degrees and points out that this acuity enables travel vision and benefits from the use of optical systems and TV magnification.

IV. Offers a new definition of those who are classified as partially seeing — that is, 10/200 to 20/60 or better acuity with restricted field of less than twenty degrees diameter. In this category, large print and optical aids are recommended.

Classification of Impaired Vision

DIAGNOSTIC AND FUNCTIONAL
Based on Optimal Visual Correction with
Standard Lenses for Better Eye

DIAGNOSTIC GROUPING	FUNCTIONAL GUIDELINES
I. Blindness	I. Braille use
A. No light perception	A. Braille dog cane and/or device wherein lack of vision is not a deterrent optical to sensory conversion
B. Light perception and projection	B. Braille cane and/or device wherein lack of vision is not a deterrent
C. Central acuity up to hand	C. Braille and/or device wherein

movements and with gross field loss

II. Hand movements to 2/200 with restricted field

III. Central acuity 2/200 up to 10/200 with form field exceeding 20°

IV. 10/200 to 20/60, or better acuity with restricted field (less than 20° diameter)

lack of vision is not a deterrent

II. Marginal form vision — assistance of light localization

III. Travel vision — use of optical systems and T.V. magnification

IV. Partially seeing; large print optical aid

NOTE: Patients with any of the above classifications of visual loss could benefit from reader service, talking books, tapes, and recordings.

The definition of legal blindness is: "A person whose central acuity does not exceed 20/200 in the better eye with corrected lenses or whose visual acuity is greater than 20/200 but is accompanied by a limitation in the field such that the widest diameter of the visual field subtends an angle of no greater than 20 degrees."

In all four groupings, however, it is pointed out that any of the persons could benefit from reader service, talking books, tapes, and recordings — important additional resources for the visually impaired.

We present these guidelines because we are the National Association for Visually Handicapped (NAVH), the only non-profit, national organization devoted solely to the field of the partially seeing. NAVH is recognized by the American Medical Association as a voluntary health agency.

The latest available statistics developed by the American Foundation for the Blind, Inc. estimate that there are approximately 6,400,000 persons in the United States whose visual impairment limits them in seeing, even with optimal corrective lenses.[1] Of these, an estimated 1,700,000 are severely impaired. This means that they are either "legally blind" or function as if they were "legally blind." The National Society for the Prevention of Blindness estimates that there are 478,800 "legally blind" in the United States with over 75 percent having some residual vision (less than 120,000 are totally blind).[2] For the remaining group of approximately 6,300,000 partially seeing individuals, NAVH has been the pioneer in the field of large print materials and we are the largest source of volunteer produced large print books in the world. Since our inception in

1954, we have produced over 120,000 volumes of 425 titles which are distributed free anywhere upon request. We act as consultants to commercial publishers to encourage them to enter this neglected field. Those who have met our standards carry the NAVH Seal of Approval which is recognized as the "mark of merit" indicating high quality publications.

Large print, although helpful for many, is only a partial answer for the visually impaired. We, therefore, cooperate with commercial manufacturers in field testing optical aids to help determine those best suited to meet the needs of the partially seeing, and NAVH serves as a continual source of information on all types of optical magnification and devices.

Being aware of the enormity of the problem of the partially seeing, NAVH has pioneered programs geared toward meeting various needs of partially seeing youngsters and their parents.

Youth groups have been conducted for young people from ages six to twenty-one. These programs have been geared to offer the visually handicapped boy and girl an opportunity to engage in social, recreational, and educational activities with normally sighted peers. For the teenager, "rap" sessions enable these young people to discover their strengths and resources which often lie beneath the surface. It is our hope that all partially seeing young people, through the programs designed to meet their specific needs, will enter an adulthood in which vocational achievement and self-fulfillment will be possible.

For the past ten years, under the leadership of professionals, parent discussion groups have been conducted. At these meetings, we orient and educate parents of the partially seeing child to help them meet the specific needs of young people with visual handicaps. We cope with the strong tendency of parents to overprotect these children — almost immobilizing them.

From the information derived through these significant sessions, NAVH has developed a family and a professional guide on the growth and development of the partially seeing child. These publications have brought comfort and understanding for thousands throughout the United States, Canada, and many foreign countries.

For the senior citizen, NAVH large type has brought pleasure and reassurance in again being able to read the printed page. Inquiries concerning services available for the older partially seeing population are answered daily. Discussion groups for the adult children of these visually impaired aged are in the process of being arranged to achieve better understanding and acceptance of the problem.

Professional education is a major concern of this agency. Many strides have been made in reaching ophthalmologists throughout the country. This year will be the twenty-first consecutive year that our agency's services will be displayed, upon invitation, in the Scientific Section of the American Academy of Ophthalmology and Otolaryngology.

Public awareness of the field of the partially seeing is vital in order to reach those who require assistance. TV and radio spots are being developed for a major educational campaign.

In order to serve the partially seeing effectively, a clearinghouse of agencies and individuals offering services is being planned. We are aware that there are many agencies that have limited services available for partially seeing people. These are mainly agencies for the blind. Since NAVH is the only national organization dedicated solely to the welfare of the partially seeing, we must serve as a referral on all available services and resources.

In order to help other agencies prevent unnecessary duplication of programs so that funds for the partially seeing may be used more effectively, we will serve as a clearinghouse. Therefore, when new money becomes available, innovative and non-duplicative programming can be developed. This is one of our goals, an extremely important one especially as funds become scarce.

As a national referral agency, our ability to achieve objectives is dependent upon the input we receive from professionals on the scene, such as ophthalmologists and rehabilitation practitioners. The interchange between NAVH and the professional community will create a new vitality within the area of service to partially seeing people — helping them achieve greater participation in the mainstream of society.

References

1. American Foundation for the Blind: *Facts About Blindness.* New York, Am Foun Blind, February 1, 1975, p. 5.
2. National Society for the Prevention of Blindness: *Annual Up-date on Estimated Total Cases and New Cases of Legal Blindness in the United States, 1975.* New York, National Society for the Prevention of Blindness, January 1976.

CHAPTER 9

TACTILE VISION SUBSTITUTION SYSTEM — APPLICATIONS TO REHABILITATION*

PAUL BACH-Y-RITA

Introduction

BLINDNESS is almost always due to loss of function of the eye, rarely is it due to brain damage. Yet we see with our brain; the eye is the camera that captures optical images, but these images are carried to the brain for interpretation. Visual responses and perception result from brain processing of the optical information delivered to it by its camera, the eye. Thus, an intriguing question arises: What would occur if an artificial eye, or camera, carried the optical information to the brain? Could blind persons then have access to visual information?

For the past twelve years a research team at the Smith-Kettlewell Institute of Visual Sciences has been studying this question. Many practical and theoretical problems have been confronted. Our results have been extensively reported elsewhere. [1-12] Portions of a recent paper have been reproduced here with permission.[7] This report will briefly review and evaluate our results, and speculate on possible future developments.

We, and other research workers in this field, e.g. Bliss,[8] have used the skin as the human sensory system to carry the visual information from the artificial eye (TV camera) to the brain. The skin is accessible, with large expanses available to our arrays of stimulators. The skin handles information in a

*This research was supported by Social and Rehabilitation Service Grant No. 14-P-55282; Research Career Development Award No. EY-14,094; The Seeing Eye, Inc., The Max C. Fleischmann Foundation, and The Smith-Kettlewell Eye Research Foundation.

manner comparable to the retina. In both cases, information is displayed in two spatial dimensions plus time. Thus even the eye is forced to carry three-dimensional information through a two-dimensional surface. The eye is, of course, far superior to the skin in its ability to simultaneously transmit many details. However, our studies have shown that a significant amount of visual information can be carried to the brain through the skin, and that the brain can be taught to interpret and use this information as "vision." Our studies are now centering on the possibility that this information can be of practical use for educational, vocational, and mobility tasks.

INSTRUMENTATION

The numerous problems and studies related to the development of comfortable, practical sensory substitution systems have been thoroughly discussed elsewhere.[5,6] The man-machine interface (the contact skin in this case) has always posed the major problem for rehabilitation engineering. We are using three types of interface: (1) an array of vibrotactile stimulators that mechanically deliver an image on the skin, (2) an array of electrical stimulators that deliver the image in the form of brief, pain-free electrical impulses, and (3) a water-jet stimulator that traces the image on the skin through a thin rubber membrane that serves to keep the subjects dry and to recirculate the water.

Considerable manipulation of the TV camera is required to meet the need for scanning or sequential exploration of a form or object. Thus the first step in training a naive blind subject to use the TVSS is the teach him to control the camera. This includes learning manual control of the aperture and focus, direction of the camera toward one or another part of the surroundings, and adjustment of the zoom lens or replacement of the interchangeable lens for close-up or distance. The hands and arms are used to move the camera with our early fixed mechanical system. With the portable system the camera is mounted on the frame of a pair of glasses; head movements are used to scan the visual field.

Having achieved familiarity with manipulation of the camera, the subject is then taught to discriminate individual lines (vertical, horizontal, diagonal, or curved) and, subsequently, combinations of lines (circles, squares, or triangles) and solid geometric forms. When these can be identified readily, a number of common objects (cup, chair, telephone) are presented in varying positions and at different distances from the camera. As the appearance of these objects becomes familiar, the blind subject discovers visual concepts such as shape distortion as a function of viewpoint and apparent change in size as a function of distance.

When two or more objects are presented simultaneously, the blind subject learns to recognize each from minimal or partial cues. Ultimately he is able to describe the layout of three or four objects on a table in correct relationship, even though they may overlap or are only partly visible. As training continues, techniques of visual analysis are developed. Indeed, our studies with the TVSS have revealed rapid perceptual learning in spite of the poor resolution of the stimulus display. New perceptual concepts, such as the perceptual use of parallax, shadows, looming, and monocular cues of depth, are learned within suprisingly few trials, although not previously experienced by the congenitally blind subjects.

Facility in directing the camera is accompanied by a change in the sensation derived from the patterned punctate stimulation of the skin. In the early stages of training (or when the camera is either immobile or under the control of another person), the subjects report experiences in terms of feeling on the area of skin which is receiving the stimuli. However, when they can easily direct the camera at will, their reports are in terms of objects localized externally in space in front of them. The provision of a motor linkage (camera movement) for the sensory receptor surface on the skin produces a surrogate "perceptual organ." The receptor surface thus becomes part of a perceptual organ which can substitute the normal visual perceptual organ, consisting of the eye with its receptors surface (the retina) and its motor apparatus (eye and neck muscles).

Neural Mechanisms Pertinent to Sensory Substitution

The ability of one sensory system to convey information normally mediated by another (lost) sensory system is dependent on the existence of plastic neural mechanisms. Evidence that brain pathways are not fixed and immutable is available from many sources. These include studies of recovery of function following brain lesions, of changes in individual neurons during learning, of alterations in evoked potentials, and of assessment of cortical structure and chemistry during sensory deprivation or enrichment. With advances in modern technology, the plastic mechanisms which permit the brain to respond to new functional requirements and to training may provide the adaptability necessary for compensating for sensory losses.

In many sensory substitution systems, including our own, an area of skin is utilized to relay the output of an artificial receptor to the brain. Large, readily accessible, and relatively flat areas of skin are available for display of an array of stimulators. The skin has numerous sensitive end organs or receptors which can respond rapidly to different types of stimulation. The dense distribution of these receptors permits the subject to make precise discriminations. Like the retina, the skin receptor surface can mediate displays in two spatial dimensions; it also has the potential for temporal integration. Three-dimensional information can be relayed through the skin for central nervous system (CNS) processing in "visual" terms. There is thus no need for complex topographical transformation or for temporal coding of pictorial information presented to the skin. Further, being a sense organ, the skin is already liberally supplied with pathways to conduct sensory information from its receptors up the spinal cord (or through the cranial nerves) to the midbrain, thalamus, and cortex.

Cutaneous receptors differ in type and distribution from one area of skin to another. However, this does not appear to pose a problem in the ability to perceive pictorial or written material displayed on the skin. Thus, our trained blind subjects can readily transfer their perception of pictorial inputs when either the type of stimulus is changed or the stimulus matrix is moved to a new area of skin.[9] Further, they are able to compensate for camera tilt even though this tilts or distorts the pattern applied to their skin. This adaptability indicates that the interpretation of a skin input as "visual" depends on plasticity of the higher regions of the CNS rather than at the peripheral level.

The TVSS places certain demands on the nervous system — the skin must assume the role of a relay rather than a receptor organ, and the higher centers are asked to process sensory information received through normal visual channels. There are a number of physiological mechanisms available to meet these demands; these have been discussed in detail elsewhere.[2,3]

The presence of plastic neural mechanisms capable of adapting to a new or artificial source of sensory information has been a key postulate in the development of a TVSS. Some of the plastic neuronal mechanisms can be altered or developed with adequate training. We have found that blind subjects learning to use a TVSS must undergo a rather specific and extensive sequence of training if they are to achieve success with the instrument. Further, an analysis of the studies of newly sighted adults who have had their vision restored surgically, after years or a lifetime of blindness,[10,11] emphasizes the need for extensive training before the subjects can learn to use their eyes to see. For example, the perceptual habits and strategies must be changed from touching to seeing. Indeed while some patients were able to see quite well shortly after surgery, possibly due to some form of self-training, others never did learn to see.

All in all, it appears easier for a blind subject to learn to use the TVSS to "see" than for the newly sighted patient to learn to use his "new" sensory input. One reason for this may be the simplicity of displays for the TVSS, in contrast to the detail and clutter of the surroundings for the newly sighted. Further, the blind subjects using the TVSS utilize a well-developed sensory input system, whereas the newly sighted use a system which may be inadequately developed or even subject to some degree of disuse atrophy at the levels of the retina, the lateral geniculate, and the cortex. It may be easier for the blind subject to expand existing mechanisms for the skin to cope with extra skin stimulators than for the newly sighted to develop or create new mechanisms to fully utilize their visual input. A final significant difference between blind subjects with the TVSS and newly sighted persons may be related to the extent to which each must accept the new "visual" input. The newly sighted have to acknowledge and adapt to a totally new status in all their endeavors. In contrast, to appreciate and utilize the TVSS, our blind subjects must recognize that it is not a replacement for their normal sensory inputs, but rather it is to provide them with a tool for certain rather specific tasks — it represents a supplement or augmentation more than a substitution.

Applications of the TVSS

One true measure of the success of any sensory aid is its practical applicability. How many handicapped persons will actually *use* it? By this criterion, the TVSS is as yet at an embryonic stage of development. With our present relatively crude apparatus, the blind subject using the TVSS does so in the controlled conditions of the uncluttered laboratory and with unlimited time for repeated scanning of an object or form. Recognition of the salient features in the visual field may take seconds or minutes, depending on the complexity of the material to be studied, although recognition time decreases markedly with practice. These conditions do not pose an insurmountable obstacle for certain practical applications of the TVSS for educational and vocational purposes. Indeed, we have already been able to demonstrate specific uses of the TVSS which on a broader scale may be of benefit to many blind persons. For example, a congenitally blind doctoral candidate in philosophy who was preparing a philosophical thesis which included a comparison of visual and tactual space was able to learn a great deal about visual space. His report, written following a two-week training session with the TVSS, is a clear description of the acquisition of visual capabilities.[12]

Educational

Results obtained thus far with the TVSS have demonstrated

the practicality of the system in learning. We have explored the presentation and recognition of forms, objects, letters, and graphical material (e.g. bar graphs) and the identification of geometric projections. Further, instruction on spatial perception, as in the appearance of a table or a coin seen from different angles or the localization in depth of several objects in the field of view, has provided our blind subjects with concepts not available by any other means. We are continually seeking improved methods for training blind subjects in the use of the TVSS with the aims of reducing training time and of enabling children to adapt to the use of the instrumentation.

The potential usefulness of the TVSS need not be limited to the blind. Preliminary studies with a modified version of the TVSS have demonstrated applicability for the education of sighted children with dyslexia and other learning disabilities. These studies, by Dr. Helen Shevill, have demonstrated increased letter recognition by means of the separate and simultaneous presentation of visual and tactile displays.

Vocational

Studies on vocational applications of the TVSS have only recently begun. In our laboratory, a workbench model has enabled a blind electronic engineer to obtain valuable information related to his work. For example, he is able to focus the oscilloscope and he is able to look for relations of wave forms to time, as well as observing the purity of the wave forms and analyzing amplifier wave forms as to their uniformity and distortion. With a TVSS adapter to a dissecting microscope, he is able to determine details of circuit boards and to perform real microassembly and microinspection tasks. Based on his experience to date, this engineer predicts that he, and other technically oriented blind persons, will be considerably more able to compete on the job market with a bench-mounted, simple system. This could be used for test situations (oscilloscopes, meters, etc.) or construction situations (identifying color coded wires and components, working with circuit boards and miniature components) in much the same way that sighted persons use a microscope, to be approached and used when needed but not necessarily worn at all times.

With technical refinements in the TVSS, but without a great increase in the resolution (number of stimulating points on the skin), I predict that practical applications for blind persons will be mainly in the areas of vocational uses and education. Applications in either of these fields do not require highly miniaturized, high-resolution, or flexible devices. In addition to the possibilities discussed above by our blind electronics engineer, vocational applications are foreseeable in other professions, e.g. for telephone and communication workers, assembly line workers, teachers, and craftsmen. In the educational field a blind student must have access to the same material as sighted students (printed matter, graphs, geometry, maps, spatial concepts, body image, etc.), but it is not absolutely necessary that the acquisition be as rapid as for sighted persons, nor is it essential that the sensory substitution device be completely portable. Studies with the Optacon® and with our TVSS system have demonstrated that considerable visual information can be acquired by blind persons. Therefore, it is reasonable to expect that improved teaching methods, earlier use by the blind (including blind infants), improved equipment, reduced cost, and wider acceptance of sensory substitution devices such as the Optacon and the TVSS will demonstrate the practicality of such devices. For such applications it is not necessary to develop a single multiple-purpose device, rather it is anticipated that a number of special purpose devices will be developed, each designed to fulfill a particular need.

This report has summarized some of our work to date. However, studies are continuing, in our laboratories and in collaborating laboratories in this country and abroad, to develop practical applications of the TVSS.

References

1. Bach-y-Rita, P.: Sensory plasticity: Applications to a visual substitution system. *Acta Neurol Scand, 43*:417-426, 1967.

2. Bach-y-Rita, P.: *Brain Mechanisms in Sensory Substitution.* New York, Academic Press, 1972.
3. Bach-y-Rita, P.: Sensory substitution. In Autrum, H. (Ed.): *Handbook of Sensory Physiology,* Vol. VIII. New York, Springer-Verlag, in press.
4. Bach-y-Rita, P., Collins, C. C., Saunders, F., White B., and Scadden, L.: Vision substitution by tactile image projection. *Nature 221*:963-964, 1969.
5. Collins, C. C. and Bach-y-Rita, P.: Transmission of pictorial information through the skin. *Advan Biol Med Phys 14*:285-315, 1973.
6. Collins, C. C. and Madey, J. M.: Tactile sensory replacement. *Proc San Diego Biomedical Symposium, 13,* 1974.
7. Bach-y-Rita, P.: Visual information through the skin — A tactile vision substitution system. *Trans Amer Acad Ophthal Otolaryng,* in press.
8. Bliss, J. C.: A reading machine with tactile display. In Sterling, T. D., Bering, Jr., E. A., Potlack, S. V., and Vaughn, Jr., H. G. (Eds.): *Visual Prosthesis: The Interdisciplinary Dialogue.* New York, Academic Press, 1971, pp. 259-263.
9. Scadden, L. A.: Tactile pattern recognition and body loci. *Perception, 2*:333-336, 1973.
10. Gregory, R. L. and Wallace, J. G.: *Recovery from Early Blindness — A Case Study,* Suppl. 2. Cambridge, England, Heffers, 1963, p. 46.
11. Valvo, A.: *Sight Restoration After Long-term Blindness: The Problems and Behavior Patterns of Visual Rehabilitation.* New York, Am Foun Blind, 1971, p.54.
12. Guarniero, A.: Tactile visual experience. *Perception,* in press.

CHAPTER 10

THE OPTACON®: ITS POSSIBILITIES AND LIMITATIONS

Harry J. Link

The Optacon

THE Optacon (OPtical-to-TActile-CONverter) is a direct-translation reading aid that makes it possible for a blind person to read ordinary printed material. To use the Optacon a blind person holds the miniature camera — it is about the size of a pocket knife — with the right hand and moves it along a line of print. The camera contains two tiny lamps plus phototransistors that register the intensity of light. These phototransistors produce signals that are converted by the Optacon into a pattern of vibrating reeds. If the camera is over the letter "O" the reeds will respond by forming a pattern that is like a crater with a vibration rim. Other letters will produce tactile patterns that correspond to their shapes.

The vibrating reeds produce an image on a "tactile screen" which is about an inch by one-half inch. A blind person can feel the entire array with one finger. The entire Optacon, including camera, tactile screen, and electronics, is about 2″× 6″ × 8″. The Optacon is battery operated and conveniently portable.

Although the Optacon embodies many advanced technological features, its principles of operation are not especially complex. The machine can be divided into three parts: The camera converts images of the print to be read into corresponding electrical impulses. The electronics section processes these electrical impulses and generates electrical power to drive the vibrators and other systems. The tactile array displays in vibrating form the page information transmitted by the electronics from the camera.

100

The camera functions much like a television camera in converting light to electronic impulses. Two miniature lamps in an opening, or "camera window," illuminate the material to be read. Light reflected from the page is focused by the zoom lens system onto the silicon "retina." The silicon "retina" corresponds to the "rods and cones" of the camera's "eye." It contains 144 phototransistors arranged in the same twenty-four row, six column fashion as are the tactile array and the visual display. Each phototransistor is a miniature solar cell converting the impinging light into electricity. The magnitude of the electrical signal thus generated is proportional to the intensity of the light. These 144 electrical signals contain the optical information and are transmitted by the camera cable to the electronics section.

The electronics section is contained within the main chassis of the Optacon. The electronics, together with the battery, generate the proper electrical power and timing signals to operate the camera and tactile array. The tactile array consists of 144 pins arranged in twenty-four rows and six columns like the silicon retina. If the impulse from a particular phototransistor is considered "dark," the pin in the same geometrical location is vibrated.

A vibratory pattern is thereby generated that exactly duplicates the pattern of "dark" elements of the retina. Since print is dark, this vibratory pattern closely approximates the printed letter patterns on the page material being read.

The vibrating pins protrude through holes in a curved plastic fingerplate. Inside the unit, the pins are attached to piezoelectric beams that generate the mechanical vibrations.

Several controls are used in operating the Optacon. One adjusts the magnification of the camera image to compensate for differences in the size of the type.

Another adjusts the intensity of the vibrating reeds. It functions like the volume control on a radio. A threshold adjustment knob determines what light intensity will cause the reeds to vibrate. This control compensates for differences in reflectivity of inks and papers.

A button on the back panel of the Optacon allows the battery charge to be checked. A switch there changes the circuitry so a blind person can read white letters on a black background or on a luminous display such as is found on electronic calculators.

Reading with the Optacon

Reading with the Optacon involves the integration of motor, perceptual, and cognitive skills. Initially, the student needs to become familiar with the equipment, learn to recognize letters, and develop skill in the two-hand coordination task of manipulating the camera and perceiving the corresponding images. Depending on their previous education, blind people with no previous visual experience may not know the detailed features of all upper case and lower case letters. Thus the first few days of training are devoted to these tasks.

The most difficult task, which is usually only initiated in a training course, is to develop sufficient reading speed so that the Optacon is useful to the individual and can be integrated into his normal functioning. Developing reading speed takes time because Optacon reading is a different mode of reading than most people are accustomed to. Since letters are only seen one at a time, the individual must extensively exercise his immediate memory in order to perceive words and phrases as a whole. In addition, inkprint documents are much more variable in terms of type style and format than braille which is standardized. The variety found in the "world of print" can be a surprise to a blind person and training is useful in helping him to cope with this.

Given normal capabilities and a strong desire for independent access to printed information, a blind individual can expect to be able to read from five to twenty words per minute at the end of about fifty hours of private instruction. This reading rate typically doubles within six months after the training course. This fifty hours of training could be an intensive course over nine days or it could be spread over several months. After this, the student should be able to practice independently from a teacher, with the speed of reading and the range of documents which he can handle with confidence gradually increasing. Over a period of six months to a year, some blind people have been able to achieve reading rates from forty to sixty words per minute, while others have not. The maximum reading rate achieved after several years of Optacon experience has been about eighty words per minute.

The Optacon was developed at Stanford University and Stanford Research Institute, primarily under United States government support over an eight-year period. The research prototype of the presently available model was completed in early 1971. Telesensory Systems, Inc., located in Palo Alto, California, was established to manufacture Optacons with the first units becoming commercially available in September of 1971. Since then over 650 Optacons have been disseminated throughout the world, four hundred in the United States and 250 outside of the United States. Dissemination is occurring at the rate of 40 optacons monthly.

Field Evaluations of the Optacon

Information from this field experience is now emerging which I will summarize as follows. One of the earliest field Optacon programs was initiated in the San Diego School District in October 1971. Five blind students participated in this program. They were not selected according to intelligence or proficiency in reading braille; however, all were braille readers.

All the normal alternatives to access to printed information (i.e. braille, tapes, sighted readers, etc.) were available to these participants through their school program. The Optacon program was an after-hours extracurricular activity.

All participants eventually achieved the project objectives of thirty words per minute in ornate type style. The mean speed attained was thirty-nine words per minute with a standard deviation of about thirteen words per minute. During this project the Optacon proved to be a relatively durable device; the average down time for the instrument was six hours over five months. Currently, all five original Optacons are still in use by the original participants. This use is on a sustained basis, meaning that Optacon reading has become a normal part of these students' functioning. The results of this evaluation have just been published.

A second experience with a group of Optacon users began in April of 1972 in a class of eighteen blind computer programmers in Heidelberg, Germany. This German rehabilitation institute had originally intended to provide its trainees with braille computer listings and manuals. One manual was being transcribed and the first few programs had been listed in braille when the Optacons were delivered. Within a short period of time there was no demand for braille output. The students only wanted the normal printout, if for no other reason than that they did not want to cause their future employers any extra work. They look up things in the normal manuals, analyze the error messages, find what they are looking for in the computer listings, and read the messages printed out on the console typewriter. They also use their Optacons for personal matters, such as reading mail and bank statements.

These students successfully completed their vocational training in data processing by the end of 1972. Early in 1973 all thirteen had signed employment contracts, ten of these being in private industry. All the subsequent classes of blind computer programmers at this institute have also been supplied Optacons.

Concurrent with this field experience in Germany, an Optacon evaluation was conducted in England by St. Dunstans and the Royal National Institute for the Blind under the leadership of Professor Michael Tobin of the University of Birmingham. In this evaluation, information was first obtained from a set of thirty blind adults and adolescents who participated in an initial Optacon training course. Since only ten Optacons were available in this program, the Optacons had to be time-shared over the year's duration of the program. In the later months of the program, information was obtained from seventeen of the original trainees who participated in extended training and practice.

The initial training showed that the most successful Optacon learners were, on the average, above the norm in terms of tactual discrimination ability, short-term memory capacity (letter-span), and braille reading speed; they were, in general, below the average of the whole group in age and in age at which braille was learned. Previous visual experience did not produce a significant correlation with performance in the initial training program.

From the seventeen participants in the extended training and practice, reading rates of some readers were only ten to twelve words per minute, while others were able, for short periods, to read from books of their own choice at speeds of about forty words per minute. The final result of the Tobin Study were published in early fall of 1974 in Research Bulletin No. 28 by the American Foundation for the Blind.

A similarly sized field experience has occurred in Sweden as well. The purpose of the Swedish project, conducted by Nilsson H. Marmolin, was to evaluate the Optacon reading aid, its practical use, and the effectivity of the training methods used. Here, twenty-seven blind people were trained with nine Optacons over a one-year period. Two of these people have already achieved reading rates over forty-five words per minute and at least twenty-two of this first group are considered to be successful readers. Repeated tests of the reading achievement in various situations during and after the Optacon course indicated that (1) practically all blind subjects can learn to identify printed letters and words with the Optacon, (2) the interindividual differences in reading skill are very great, (3) the practical usefulness of the Optacon is limited to certain individuals and certain situations, and (4) the Optacon training methods can be made more effective. The results of earlier investigations supported these conclusions which must be considered as preliminary as relatively few individuals have received instruction and only few have had access to an Optacon for a longer period of time. It was indicated that further investigations would focus on developing more effective instruction and training methods.

Of the field experiences in the United States, the American Institutes for Research has been conducting an education evaluation under contract with the United States Office of Education since September 1972. This study involves over fifty Optacons in about fifteen schools throughout the United States. About eighty-five blind students from fourth to twelfth grade are participating. After twenty-four class hours of training, reading rates from one to seventeen words per minute were achieved.

Some of the major conclusions stated in an interim report covering the first fifteen months of this study — to test alternative teaching arrangements, identify predictors of Optacon success, and observe the effect of Optacon training on student attitudes — are the following: (1) Blind elementary and secondary age students can learn to use the Optacon to read standard print with high accuracy. (2) Both tutorial and small group instructional approaches are viable alternatives. (3) Intelligence (WISC and WAIS verbal scale) and tactile ability (Tactile-Kinesthetic Form Discrimination Test) are useful predictors of Optacon reading rate and accuracy and variety of use, at least during training.

The Franklin Institute Research Laboratories has evaluated the Optacon from an engineering standpoint. This was a counterpart to the AIR study under a contract with the United States Office of Education. The conclusions about the Optacon fall into two general segments — general impressions and recommended improvements. They say that "engineering studies have proven that the design (of the Optacon) is basically sound and indications suggest that it is a reliable system," and "a host of minor improvements are recommended which would optimize user convenience and minimize cost in its present configuration." However, they state that it would take considerable research and development to accomplish these recommended changes of innovations. The report also states, "Potential users, virtually unanimously, reported that the Optacon would be very useful in their daily lives."

The larger field experience in the United States has resulted from the participation of about 150 blind individuals in training classes given at about a dozen locations. From this experience, considerable knowledge of the learning process has been acquired and a five-volume training course has been developed by Telesensory Systems, Inc.

In the spring of 1973, the Richard King Mellon Foundation embarked upon a two-year project to demonstrate the utility of the Optacon to approximately 125 blind adults and children in Pittsburgh, Pennsylvania. The eight participating organizations consist of four agencies serving the blind, three school systems, and the University of Pittsburgh.

In February of 1974, the American Foundation for the Blind was requested to conduct a program impact evaluation study of the Mellon Foundation Program. The primary purposes of this study were to evaluate the effectiveness of the Optacon training programs of the participating agencies and to assess the accomplishments and experiences of the Optacon trainees. This study was completed in July of 1975.

Criteria for Reading Machines

Previous research on reading machines for the blind has indicated four general criteria for such a machine to be considered useful. First, the reading machine must read printed material directly, and there could be no compromise on this point. That is, if any form of special treatment must be administered in the printing process or if the print had to be translated in any way prior to its use in the machine, then the purpose of the reading machine was defeated without any further consideration. A reading machine must be capable of reading the same print available to the sighted population. Second, the reading machine should be portable. Third, the machine should be reasonable in cost. (Definition of reasonable cost ranged from figures of $300 or $400 per unit by sighted people, up to estimates of $1200 made by blind persons.) The fourth criterion was the machine's usefulness to blind people in strictly a reading sense. That is, the blind person should be able to read with the machine at a rewarding rate after a reasonable amount of training. A rewarding rate meant many things to many people. To some blind people it meant 2 words per minute; to an authority in the field it meant 100 words per minute for the average, well-trained user, with optimum speeds of perhaps 200 words per minute and absolute minimum speeds of 50 to 60 words per minute. In general, estimates of a minimum reading speed for a successful reading machine were in the neighborhood of 20 words per minute.

How does the Optacon compare with these four criteria — keeping in mind that criteria do change, especially as blind people become more experienced in the usage of a reading machine?

The Optacon does not require any special processing or translation with regard to printed material. The only requirement on the print is that it be within a certain size range which is between six point and twenty point, this point range includes about 95 percent of the material in print. The versatility of material which can be read is limited only by the perceptual and interpretive abilities of the reader.

The present Optacon is completely portable, carried in a small leather case with a shoulder strap. It operates on batteries or AC current.

The Optacon's major drawback, however, is its cost which is $3,450. In addition, about fifty hours of Optacon training is necessary. Training is provided at several locations — either at Telesensory Systems, Inc. in Palo Alto, California, the manufacturer of the Optacon, or at one of fifteen training centers established in the United States. The cost of training at TSI is $500.00. The cost in the other training centers may range from no cost up to $500 depending on the student's financial situation. The decision to purchase the Optacon is generally made upon completion of training.

While the price is substantial, it appears reasonable in view of the cost of manufacturing in relatively small lot sizes plus the cost of proper engineering, support, service, and marketing. It is anticipated that with increased production the cost will be reduced.

Reading speed has been of particular interest in the scientific evaluations of the Optacon, yet, according to the AFB report "The Optacon: A Valuable Device for the Blind" by Goldish and Taylor, almost eighty of the one hundred users interviewed by telephone indicated that reading speed is not of primary importance. Comments such as, "If I read only two words per minute, this would still be better than before I got my Optacon." and "Even if I could read only a few words per minute, I could still find use for my Optacon." were common. Nevertheless, most users indicated that some minimum speed — perhaps fifteen to twenty words per minute — is necessary for the device to be useful; comprehension is said to suffer at very slow reading rates. Reading speed was cited as being of importance primarily by those who must read voluminous material with the Optacon.

A blind individual can expect to be able to read from five to twenty words per minute at the end of about fifty hours of private instruction. This reading rate may double within six months after the training course. Reading rates appear to increase with Optacon experience and with practice. Reading speeds between eighty and one hundred words per minute were reported, although indications are that a typical Optacon user, with adequate practice, might expect to achieve a nominal speed of between thirty and sixty words per minute. Actual reading speed varies with quality of print, complexity of content, personal interest, and level of reader fatigue. The Optacon reading rates usually are considerably slower than the braille reading rates of users who read braille regularly — typically about one third as fast.

When asked to describe the most significant advantages of the Optacon, over half the users sited independence, the ability to read without relying on an intermediary such as a braillist or a reader, as the primary value of the Optacon. Accessibility to the printed word was sited next often, followed by immediacy, the ability to read material when and where desired. Other values of significant importance include the ability to read material in privacy and the portability of the Optacon. The true utility of the Optacon, however, is highly subjective; it depends upon the needs and aspirations of the user.

Optacon Usage

From an employment standpoint the Optacon seems to be particularly suited in a number of situations. To what extent the Optacon will open new job opportunities for the blind requires further exploration since most of the blind people who have received Optacon training were employed prior to training.

The Optacon is particularly suited for use by blind computer professionals since computer output has a standard format, a computer user knows his own program, and the vocabulary of the programming language is limited. Many computer professionals indicate that although reading braille is much faster and requires less effort than reading with an Optacon, the Optacon may eliminate the need in some situations for special print-out and, in the long run, reduces program turn-around time.

Data processors are using the Optacon for reading sections of computer manuals, for reviewing segments of extensive print-outs, and for analyzing error messages. Programmers indicate that the Optacon allows them to examine print-outs and other materials in their actual format. Thus, they are aware of columnar structure, positions of headings, and overall layout.

Some lawyers use their Optacons to read the shorter, more concise legal materials such as law statues, judicial opinions, and journal articles.

Some engineers use their Optacons to read technical journals and reference books, very few of which are available in braille or on tape. The Optacon also enables the engineers to read graphs and schematic diagrams, the maplike line representations of electronic and logic circuits.

From an educational viewpoint, the Optacon enables a blind student to have access to critical material when he needs it. With the proper accessories, it enables the student to read computer terminal print-outs and to utilize electric pocket calculators which facilitate success in the math and computer courses which many blind students are choosing. For the younger student, the Optacon can be utilized for the development of a sighted perspective to rather difficult material such as math and science, enhancing learning of these subjects.

In terms of daily living, the privacy and personal independence which the machine makes possible for a blind person is invaluable. Independent management of personal finances, private written communication with sighted friends, and organization of personal papers and records are possible when the blind person can read print with the Optacon.

Extensions of the Optacon Concept

The basic Optacon instrument with slight modifications can be used for reading tasks other than normal reading. These other applications may prove to significantly extend the capabilities of a blind person and to open up new educational and vocational opportunities.

For example, an Optacon accessory lens is available which enables the visual display on many electronic calculators to be read. The importance of this accessory is that it enables a blind person to make computations to ten place accuracy involving nonlinear functions — a capability that is virtually impossible by any other portable means without sighted help.

In addition, another modification is possible which enables many video terminals to be read with the Optacon. The cathode ray tube, or television tube, is becoming an increasingly popular information display device and is employed in airline reservation offices, customer service centers, as well as computation centers. The capability of a blind person to read such terminals not only expands opportunity for employment but protects against obsolescence for computer programmers. Optacon accessories are also planned which will aid a blind person in typing and handwriting.

Conclusion

The information from various field experiences seems to strongly indicate that the Optacon can play an important function for some blind individuals. It appears to be an effective tool in its present form for people who are able and are motivated to master the skills required to use it. Moreover, various accessories are available, or are becoming available, which may extend the Optacon's range of usefulness, particularly in specialized areas.

More effective Optacon-like tools may be possible if further research efforts are made. Initial investigations at Stanford University on a "next generation" Optacon have produced some interesting results indicating the feasibility of significant improvements. These investigations were on a "one-hand Optacon" which would incorporate the camera and tactile array in one unit. A functional simulation of this new configuration has been constructed and reading tests are being conducted to ascertain what performance improvement results, if any. At this time, we can only say that current Optacon users have been able to match their Model R-1B reading rates with the "one-hand" version in a matter of a few hours. Thus there seems to be no obsolescence problem, in that a good Optacon user with presently available equipment will essentially be trained for this form of "next generation."

References

Baer, James A. and Hill, John W.: *Optical-to-Tactile Image Conversion for the Blind*. HEW, Social and Rehabilitation Service, final report on Contract SRS 70-42 and Grant 14-P-55296/9-02. Menlo Park, California, Stanford Research Institute, June 1972.

Bliss, James C., Katcher, Michael H., Rogers, Charles H., and Shepard, Raymond P.: Optical-to-tactile image conversion for the blind. *IEEE Transactions on Man-Machine Systems*, MMS-11(1), March 1970.

Calhoun, C. Robert, Lutz, Gale W., and Knab, Karen: *San Diego Optacon Project 1971-1972*. San Diego, California, San Diego Unified School District, July 1972.

Coffey, John L. and McFarland, Ray R.: *The Evaluation and Standardization of Selection and Training Procedures for the Battelle Aural Reading Device*. Submitted to Veterans Administration, final report on Contract No. V1005 M-1961. June 1963.

Goldish, R. H. and Taylor, H. E.: The Opatcon: A valuable device for blind persons. *New Outlook for the Blind*, February 1974. Telesensory Systems, Inc.: Teaching Guidelines (R17454-B). Palo Alto, California, Telesensory Systems, Inc., 1974.

Tobin, M. J., James, W. R. K., McVeigh, A., and Irving, R. M.: *Print Reading by the Blind — An Evaluation of the Optacon and an Investigation of Some Learner Variables and Teaching Methods*. Birmingham, England, Research Centre for the Education of the Visually

Handicapped, School of Education, University of Birmingham, 1973.

Weisgerber, Robert A., Everett, Bruce E., Rodabaugh, Barbara J., Shanner, William M., Crawford, Jack J.: *Educational Evaluation of the Optacon (Optical-to-Tactile Converter) as a Reading Aid to Blind Elementary and Secondary Students,* AIR-34500-9/74-FR. Submitted to the U.S. Office of Education, Bureau of Education for the Handicapped, final report on Contract No. OEC-0-72-5180. Washington, D. C., September 1974.

Willson, G. T.: *The Royal National Institute for the Blind International Survey of Optacon Users — Part I, June 3rd-22nd, 1974.* Unpublished report.

CHAPTER 11

VOCATIONAL REHABILITATION OF THE BLIND AND SEVERELY VISUALLY IMPAIRED*

JOHN G. CULL AND RICHARD E. HARDY

Psychological Adjustment to Blindness

IT is true that our clients are much more like us than unlike us, but they differ in one major respect. They have suffered the psychological impact of disability and have adjusted or are in the process of adjusting to this impact. In this chapter we shall discuss the factors which affect the psychological adjustment to blindness and the mechanism by which an individual adjusts to his blindness.

During the first and second world wars, behavioral scientists noticed an increased incidence in conversion reactions. Conversion reactions are (APA, 1965) a type of psychoneurotic disorder in which the impulse causing anxiety is *converted* into functional symptoms in parts of the body rather than the anxiety being experienced consciously. Examples of conversion reactions include such functional disabilities as anesthesias (blindness, deafness), paralyses (aphonia, monoplegia, or hemiplegia), dyskineses (tic, tremor, catalepsy).

The study of these conditions along with other studies led to the development of a discipline known as psychosomatic medicine. Psychosomatic medicine is concerned with the study of the effects of the personality and emotional stresses upon the body and its function. This psychological interaction with physiology can be observed in any of the body systems.

*From Richard E. Hardy and John G. Cull, *Severe Disabilities: Social and Rehabilitation Approaches*, 1975. Courtesy of Charles C Thomas, Publisher, Springfield, Illinois.

After establishment of psychosomatic medicine, behavioral scientists (psychiatrists, psychologists, social workers, etc.) began observing the converse of this new field. Instead of studying the effects of emotional stress on bodily functioning, they studied the effects of physical stress on emotional functioning. Their concern was directed toward answering the question, "What are the emotional and personality changes which result from physical stress or a change in body function or physical configuration?"

Role of Body-image in Adjustment to Blindness

This new area of study became known as somatopsychology. The basis for this study is the body-image concept. The body-image is a complex conceptualization which we use to describe ourselves. It is one of the basic parts of the total personality and as such determines our reaction to our environment. According to English and English (1966) the body-image is the mental representation one has of his own body.

There are two aspects of the body-image concept — the ideal body-image (the desired body-image) and the actual body-image. The greater the congruity between these two images the better the psychological adjustment of the individual, and conversely, the greater the discrepancy between these two parts of the self-concept, the poorer an individual's psychological adjustment. This is very understandable. If an individual is quite short and views himself as such but has a strong ideal body-image of a tall person, he is less well adjusted than he would be if his desired image were that of a short person. This is a simplistic example, but it portrays the crux of the psychological adjustment to blindness.

In order to adjust to the psychological impact of blindness, the body-image has to change from the image of a sighted person to the body-image of a blind person. Early in the adjustment process the actual body-image will change from that of a sighted person to the actual body-image of a blind person; however, for adequate psychological adjustment to the blindness the ideal body-image must make the corresponding adaptation. Therefore, in essence, psychological adjustment to a disability is the acceptance of an altered body-image which is more in harmony with reality.

Factors Associated with Adjustment

There are three groups of factors which determine the speed or facility with which an individual will adjust to his disability. They help an individual understand the degree of psychological impact a particular disability is having on a client and the significance of his adjustment.

The first of these three groups of factors are those directly associated with the disability. Psychological effects of disabilities may arise from direct insult or damage to the central nervous system. These psychological effects are called brain syndromes and may be either acute or chronic. In disabilities involving no damage to brain tissue the physical limitations imposed by the disability may cause excessive frustration and in turn result in behavioral disorders. For example, an active outdoorsman and nature lover may experience a greater psychological impact upon becoming blind than an individual who leads a more restricted and physically limited life since the restrictions imposed by the disability demand a greater change in the basic life-style of the first person. Therefore, factors directly associated with the disability have an important bearing upon an individual's reaction to disability.

The second group consists of those factors arising from the individual's attitude toward his disability. An individual's adjustment to his disability is dependent upon the attitudes he had prior to his disability. If his attitudes toward the blind were quite negative and strong he will naturally have a greater adjustment problem than an individual with a neutral or positive attitude toward disability and the disabled, or, specifically, the blind and blindness. A part of this attitude formation prior to blindness is dependent upon the experiences the client had with other blind individuals and the stereotypes he developed.

The amount of fear a client experiences or the emotion he expends during the onset and duration of the illness or accident leading up to the disability will determine the psychological impact of the disability. Generally, the greater the amount of emotion expended during onset the better the psychological adjustment to the disability. If an individual goes to sleep a sighted person and awakens a blinded person, his psychological reaction to the disability is much greater than if a great deal of emotion is expended during a process of becoming blinded.

The more information an individual has relating to his disability the less impact the disability will have. If the newly blinded individual is told about his blindness in a simple, straight-forward, mechanistic manner, it is much easier to accept and adjust to the disability than if it remains shrouded in a cloak of ignorance and mystery. Any strangeness or unpredictable aspect of our body associated with its function immediately creates anxiety and if not clarified rapidly can result in totally debilitating anxiety. Therefore, it is important for psychological adjustment to a disability that the individual have communicated to him, in terms he can understand, the medical aspects of his disability as soon after onset of the disability as possible.

When we are in strange or uncomfortable surroundings, our social perceptiveness becomes keener. Social cues which are below threshold or are not noticed in comfortable surroundings become highly significant to us in new, strange, or uncomfortable surroundings. Upon the onset of blindness, the client will develop a heightened perceptiveness relative to how he is being treated by family, friends, and professionals. If others start treating him in a condescending fashion and relegate him to a position of less importance, his reaction to the psychological impact of the blindness will be poor. Professionals can react to the client from an anatomical orientation (what is missing) or a functional orientation (what is left). The anatomical orientation is efficient for classification purposes but is completely dehumanizing. The functional orientation is completely individualistic and, as such, enhances a client's adjustment to his disability.

Perhaps a key concept in the adjustment to blindness is the evaluation of the future and the individual's role in the future. In many physical medicine rehabilitation centers, a rehabilitation counselor is one of the first professionals to see the patient after the medical crisis has passed. The purpose of this approach is to facilitate the patient's psychological adjustment. If he feels there is a potential for his regaining his independence and security the psychological impact of the blindness will be lessened. While the counselor cannot engage in specific vocational counseling with the patient, he can discuss the depth of the vocational rehabilitation program and through these preliminary counseling sessions the counselor can help the newly blinded person evaluate the roles he might play in the future.

The last factor which determines the adjustment process is based upon the individual's view of the purpose of his body and the relationship this view has with the type and extent of disability. The views individuals have of their body may be characterized as falling somewhere on a continuum. At one end of the continuum is the view that the body is a tool to accomplish work; it is a productive machine. At the other end is the view that the body is an esthetic stimulus to be enjoyed and provide pleasure for others. This latter concept is much the same as we have for sculpture and harks back to the philosophy of the ancient Greeks. Everyone falls somewhere on this continuum. To adequately predict the impact of a disability upon an individual, one has to locate the placement of the individual upon this continuum and then evaluate the disability in the light of the individual's view of the function of this body.

As an example of the above principle, consider the case in which a day laborer and a film actress sustain the same disabling injury — a deep gash across the face. Obviously, when considering the disability in conjunction with the assumed placements of these two upon the functional continuum, the psychological impact will be greater for the actress; since we have assumed the day laborer views his body almost completely as a tool to accomplish work and the disability has not impaired that function; the psychological impact of the disability upon him will be minimal. However, if the disability were changed (they both sustained severe injury to the abdomen resulting in the destruction of the musculature of the abdominal wall) the psychological impact would be reversed. In this case the actress would view her disability as minimal since it did not interfere with the esthetic value of her body, while the day laborer's disability would be over-powering since it had substantial effects upon the productive capacity of his body.

The most obvious conclusion to be drawn from the above three factors is that the degree of psychological impact is not correlated with the degree of disability. This statement is contrary to popular opinion; however, disability and its psychological impact constitute a highly personalized event. Many counselors fall into the trap of equating degree of disability with degree of psychological impact. If the psychological impact suffered by a client is much greater than that considered *normal*, the counselor will oftentimes become impatient with the client. It should be remembered that relatively superficial disabilities may have devastating psychological effects. The psychological impact of total blindness is not necessarily greater than partial blindness or, for that matter, more anatomically superficial physical disabilities.

Role of Defense Mechanisms in Adjustment

While the three groups of factors discussed above determine the length of time required for adjustment to blindness, the path to adjustment is best described by defense mechanisms. Defense mechanisms are psychological devices used by all to distort reality. Often reality is so harsh it is unacceptable to us. Therefore, we distort the situation to make it more acceptable. Defense mechanisms are used to satisfy motives which cannot be met in reality; they reduce tensions in personal interactions; and they are used to resolve conflicts. To be effective they must be unconscious. They are not acquired consciously or deliberately. If they become conscious they become ineffective as defenses and others must replace them. For the major part of the remainder of this chapter we will look at the defenses most often employed by the disabled in the general order of their use.

Denial

Denial is an unconscious rejection of an obvious fact which is too disruptive of the personality or too emotionally painful to accept. Therefore, in order to soften reality the obvious fact is denied. Immediately upon onset of disability the individual denies it happened. Then, as the fact of the disability becomes so overwhelming its existence can no longer be denied, there is a denial of the permanency of the disability. The newly blinded individual, while utilizing the defense of denial, will adamantly maintain that he shall see again. There will be a miraculous cure or a new surgical technique will be discovered.

While there are few steadfast rules in human behavior, one is that rehabilitation, at best, can be only marginally successful at this point. Rehabilitation cannot proceed adequately until the client accepts the permanency of the disability and is ready to cope with the condition. This is what is meant by many professionals when they say a client must accept his blindness. Most clients will never accept their blindness, but they should and will accept the permanence of the blindness. Denial is the front line of psychological defense but it may outlast all other defenses.

Withdrawal

Withdrawal is a mechanism which is used to reduce tension by reducing the requirements for interaction with others within the individual's environment. There are two dynamics which result from withdrawal. In order to keep from being forced to face the acceptance of the newly acquired blindness, the individual withdraws. As a result of the client's changed physical condition — blindness — his social interaction is quite naturally reduced. His circle of interest as determined by friends, business, social responsibilities, church, civic responsibilities, and family is drastically reduced. Thus, the client becomes egocentrically oriented until finally his entire world revolves around himself.

Rather than functioning interdependently with his environment to mutually fulfill needs as our culture demands, he is concerned exclusively with his environment fulfilling his needs. As his world becomes more narrowed, his thoughts and preoccupations become more somatic. Physiological processes heretofore unconscious now become conscious. At this point he begins using another defense mechanism — regression.

Regression

Regression is the defense mechanism which reduces stress by avoiding it. The individual psychologically returns to an earlier age that was more satisfying. He adopts the type of behavior that was effective at that age but now has been outgrown and substituted by more mature behavior — behavior which is more effective in coping with stressful situations.

As the newly blinded individual withdraws, becomes egocentric, and hypochrondriacal, he will regress to an earlier age which was more satisfactory. This regression may be manifested in two manners. First, he may, in his regression, adopt the dress, mannerisms, speech, etc. of the contemporaries at the age level to which he is regressing. Second, he may adopt the outmoded dress, mannerisms, speech, etc. of the age to which he regressed. This second manifestation of regression is considerably more maladaptive since it holds the individual out to more ridicule which, at this point in his adjustment to his blindness, quite possibly will result in more emphasis on the defense mechanism of withdrawal.

While utilizing the first three defense mechanisms, if reality is being harshly pushed on him and his defenses are not working, he may, as a last resort, become highly negative of those around him and negative in general. This negativism is demonstrated as an active refusal, stubbornness, contradictory attitudes, and rebellion against external demands. He may become abusive of those around and may become destructive in an effort to act out the thwarting he is experiencing. This negativisic behavior is an indication that the defense mechanisms he is employing are not distorting reality enough to allow him to adjust to his newly acquired disabled status. If, however, he is able to adjust and the defense mechanisms are effective to this point, he will employ the next defense.

Repression

Repression is selective forgetting. It is contrasted with suppression which is a conscious, voluntary forgetting. Repression is unconscious. Events are repressed because they are psychologically traumatic. As mentioned above, the attitudes the client had relative to blindness and the blinded has a major bearing upon his adjustment. If these attitudes are highly negative the client will have to repress them at this point if his adjustment is to progress. Until he represses them he will be unable to accept the required new body-image.

Reaction Formation

When an individual has an attitude which creates a great deal of guilt, tension, or anxiety and he unconsciously adopts the opposite of this attitude, he has developed a reaction formation. In order to inhibit a tendency to flee in terror a boy will express his nonchalance by whistling in the dark. Some timid persons, who feel anxious in relating with others, hide behind a facade of gruffness and assume an attitude of hostility to protect themselves from fear. A third and last example is that of a mother who, feeling guilty about her rejection of a newborn child, may adopt an attitude of extreme overprotectiveness to reduce the anxiety produced by this guilt of rejection. This example is seen more often in cases of parents with handicapped children.

In this new, dependent role the blinded individual will feel a varying degree of hostility and resentment toward those upon whom he is so dependent — wife, relatives, etc. Since these feelings are unacceptable he will develop a reaction formation. The manifest behavior will be marked by concern, love, affection, closeness — all to an excessive degree.

Fantasy

Fantasy is daydreaming. It is the imaginary representative of satisfactions that are not attained in real experience. This defense mechanism quite often accompanies withdrawal. As the client starts to adjust to a new body-image and a new role in life, he will develop a rich, overactive fantasy life. In this dreamworld he will place himself into many different situations to see how well he fits.

Rationalization

Rationalization is giving socially acceptable reasons for behavior and decisions. There are four generally accepted types of rationalization. The first is called blaming an incidental cause: the child who stumbles blames the stool by kicking it; the poor or sloppy workman blames his tools. Sour grapes rationalization is called into play when an individual is thwarted. A goal to which the individual aspires is blocked to him; therefore, he devalues the goal by saying he did not really want it so much. The opposite type of rationalization is called sweet lemons. When something the individual does not want is forced upon him, he will modify his attitude by saying it was really a very desirable goal and he feels quite positive about the new condition. The fourth and last type of rationalization is called the doctrine of balances. In this type of rationalization we balance positive attributes in others with perceived negative qualities. And conversely, we balance negative attributes with positive qualities. For example, beautiful women are assumed to be dumb, bright young boys are assumed to be weak and asthenic, and the poor are happier than the rich.

The blinded individual will have to rationalize his disability in order to assist himself in accepting the permanence of the blindness. One rationalization may be that he had nothing to do with his current condition, but that something over which he had no control caused the blindness. Another dynamic which might be observed is the adherence to the belief on the part of the client that as a result of the blindness there will be compensating factors. He will develop in other areas such as additional senses or aptitudes and talents he previously did not possess, e.g. an aptitude for music.

We once had a client whose rationalization of his disability ran something like this: All of the men in his family had been highly active outdoors types. They all had died prematurely with coronaries. He, the client, was a highly active outdoors type; however, now that he was severely disabled he would be considerably restricted in his activities. Therefore, he would not die prematurely. This logic resulted in the conclusion that the disability was positive and he was pleased he had become disabled. Granted, rationalization is seldom carried to this extreme in the adjustment to blindness, but this case is illustrative of a type of thinking which must occur for good adjustment.

Projection

A person who perceives traits or qualities in himself which are unacceptable may deny these traits and project them to others. In doing so he is using the defense mechanism of projection. A person who is quite stingy sees others as being essentially more stingy. A person who is basically dishonest sees others as trying to steal from him. A person who feels inferior rejects this idea and instead projects it to others, i.e. he is capable but others will not give him a chance because they doubt his ability. These are examples of projection. With the blinded person many of the feelings he has of himself are unacceptable. Therefore, in order to adjust adequately, he projects these feelings to society in general. *They* feel he is inadequate. *They* feel he is not capable. *They* feel he is inferior and is to be devalued. This type of thinking, normally, leads directly into identification and compensation which are in reality the natural exits to this maze in which he has been wandering around.

Identification

The defense mechanism of identification is used to reduce an individual's conflicts through the achievement of another person or a group of people. Identification can be with material possessions as well as people. A person may derive his social adequacy and psychological adequacy through his clothes (*The clothes make the man.*), his sports car, his hi-fi stereo paraphernalia, etc. People identify with larger groups in order to take on the power, prestige, and respect attributed to that organization (*our team won*). This larger group may be a club, lodge, garden club, college, professional group, etc.

In adjustment to his blindness, the client will identify with a larger group. It may be a group of other blind persons, an occupational group, a men's lodge, a veteran's group, etc. But at this point in the adjustment process, he will identify with some group in order to offset some of his feelings he has as a result of the projection he is engaging in. If successful, the identification obviates the need to employ the mechanisms of denial, withdrawal, and regression.

Compensation

If an individual's path to a set of goals is blocked and he finds other routes to achieve that set of goals, he is using the defense mechanism of compensation. A teenager is seeking recognition and acceptance from his peers. He decides to gain this recognition through sports. However, when he fails to make the team he decides to become a scholar. This is an example of compensation. Compensation brings success; therefore, it diverts attentions from shortcomings and defects, thereby eliminating expressed or implied criticism. This defense mechanism is most often used to reduce self-criticism rather than external criticism. As the individual experiences successes he will become less preoccupied with anxieties relating to his disability and his lack of productivity.

Identification and compensation usually go together in the adjustment process. When a client starts using these two defenses he is at a point at which he may adequately adjust to the new body-image and his new role in life.

Implications for Professionals Working with Blind Persons

Almost everyone in our society views handicapping and disabling conditions from an anatomical point of view rather than functionally. It is imperative that the newly blinded be helped to view their disability functionally rather than anatomically. The client should gain an appreciation for the abilities he has left rather than classifying himself with a group based solely upon an anatomical loss.

The worker with the blind should make sure the information which the client has is factual, concise, and clear. He should be sure the client's perception of his disability is correct and the cause is completely understood. This understanding greatly enhances the adjustment of the client to his blindness.

The client should be helped in exploring his feelings regarding the manner in which he is currently being treated by family and friends. Help him to understand the natural emotional reactions he will have resulting from his newly acquired blindness; and help him to understand that the feelings of family and friends are going to be different for a period of time while they adjust to his disability.

Do not fall into the trap of thinking that the degree of blindness is correlated with the degree of psychological impact. Realize that each individual's disability is unique unto that individual and his reaction to his disability will be unique.

The most important role anyone can play in assisting a client in the adjustment to blindness is to be a warm, empathic, accepting individual who is positive in his regard toward the client and who is pragmatic in counseling and planning efforts with the client.

Providing Counseling Services

What Is Counseling?

Counseling has been defined in various terms and by many experts. Gustard (1953) has written that "counseling is a learning oriented process, carried on in a simple, one-to-one social environment in which a counselor, professionally competent in relative psychological skills and knowledge, seeks to assist the client to learn more about himself, to know how to put understanding into effect in relation to clearly perceived, realistically defined goals to the end that the client may become a happier and more productive member of his society."

While definitions vary according to the orientation of the counselor, certain truisms have resulted from the enormous amount of research concerning the effectiveness of counseling. These will be explained in the following paragraphs.

No matter what particular school or theory of counseling is accepted by the practitioner, the most important factor determining the outcome of counseling effectiveness is the *personality* of the counselor himself. In other words, whether he counts himself as Rogerian, Ellisonian, or eclectic, the personality of the counselor will come through in counseling sessions and affect the outcome to a degree which will determine whether or not the counseling session is effective. Just as teachers can bring about enormous growth and changes in students by modifying their attitudes toward various subject matter, the counselor can bring about substantial changes in his client for better or worse.

Effective counseling requires certain basic ingredients. As the strength or weakness of these ingredients varies so does the ability of the counselor to help the client. There are three basic prerequisites to effective counseling. First, the counselor must accept the client without imposing conditions for this acceptance. He must be willing to work with the client and become actively involved with him as an individual no matter what the counselee's race, attitudes, or mode of life may be. This is necessary in order for the counselee to gain the knowledge that the counselor as a person wishes to help him with his problems and is not prejudging.

The counselor must be *genuine* in that he must function in a way which indicates to the client that he is being true to his own feelings and to himself. To be otherwise is to present a facade to the client — a false image which will act as a deterrant to a successful relationship. Counselors must avoid artificiality in their relationships. If the counselor hides behind a professional mystique, he may find that the counselee is better at *fooling* him than he is at deceiving the client. The professional worker cannot expect his client to be open, sincere, and genuine if he himself does not represent these characteristics well.

In addition, the counselor must have an empathetic understanding and feeling *vis-à-vis* the client. He must make a sincere effort to see the client's problem through the *client's eyes* and he must be able to communicate the depth of his understanding.

Counseling can be considered a relationship between two persons which is conducive to good mental health. Inherent in an effective counseling relationship is the absence of threat. The counselor must remove threat if the client is to grow and be able to solve his problems in an uninhibited manner. Counseling as a relationship is also typified by the types of feelings that many of us have for our closest friends. True close friendships are characterized by honest caring, genuine interest, and a high level of concern about helping in a time of need. Real friendships often require one person to put aside his own selfish needs in order to listen long enough and with enough empathy so that a friend's problem may begin to work itself out in a natural and constructive manner.

There are a number of adjectives which apply to various types of counseling (religious, marital, rehabilitation, educational, personal, vocational, and others). Counseling services vary according to the needs of the client, not the counselor. A counselee who comes to the counselor for help will often, at first, outline a concern which is not the real problem. The counselor must have considerable flexibility and insight to know what is required in each individual situation.

Rehabilitation Counseling

Rehabilitation counselors are concerned mainly with individuals who have vocational handicaps. These handicaps may result from physical disability, emotional and mental illness, social or cultural deprivation. In each individual case, the counselor must be able to decide what remedy is required in order to move the counselee toward successful personal adjustment in his family, community, and on the job.

Rehabilitation counseling requires the ingredients mentioned earlier for effective counselor-client relationships; however, much of rehabilitation counseling consists of advice-giving and coordination of services to the client. In a sense, *rehabilitation counseling* can be considered a misnomer when the term is applied across the board. A substantial number of clients need considerable advice and information which the counselor has to offer concerning social and rehabilitation services from which they can profit. When the counselee needs advice and information, the rehabilitation counselor must be able to recognize this need and provide what is required. There also will be many instances in which the client and counselor must enter into a number of counseling sessions in depth. The counselor must make the judgment concerning what type of help is needed for the client to solve his particular problems. Rehabilitation counselors need appropriate training that will enable them to decide whether or not they are qualified to do the kind of counseling which is necessary.

Many counselors fall into the trap of wanting to play the role of *junior therapist* and involve high percentages of their clients in in-depth counseling sessions. This is particularly true of the graduates of many rehabilitation counselor training programs. Some workers hide behind *counseling* (as synonymous with quality) in terms of their justifying low numbers of rehabilitated clients. There is much talk of quality services and in-depth counseling which require considerable time. The rehabilitation counselor who is an effective manager of his caseload can *rehabilitate* the number of persons required by his agency administrator and while doing so can provide counseling services as needed to his clients.

Rehabilitation work requires a broad definition of counseling which includes the offering of some, and coordination of other professional services to clients. Generally, agency administrators — especially those trained in counseling — do not accept the explanation of *the time required and quality services* for a low client rehabilitation rate. Any agency administrator or supervisor knows that some cases require much involved counseling, and that these cases, in many instances, are the most difficult ones. They are time-consuming, and they can test the fiber of the rehabilitation counselor. Untrained counselors generally cannot handle such cases without help from someone who had had some advanced orientation in counseling. However, counselors who play the role of *junior therapist* in trying to become deeply involved with all of their clients — whether or not this type of service is called for — will be ineffective and probably will not remain long in rehabilitation work.

The rehabilitation counselor will find his coordinating and facilitating role highly rewarding when it is done well and gets needed services. One of the greatest satisfactions that the counselor can have is the assurance that he knows when certain types of services are required and whether these should be more therapeutically oriented or more oriented toward advice, information, and coordination of community resources and professional services.

Rehabilitation counselors should not rank-order their clients in a psychological need hierarchy which places the individual with severe psychological problems at the top of the counselor's list for services. Certainly, these persons should be served immediately upon the counselor's realization that severe psychological problems exist. They should be referred to the appropriate psychologist or psychiatrist if problems are so severe that the counselor cannot handle them alone, or they should be served by rehabilitation counselors who are competent in the type of service required. The point to be made here is that the rehabilitation process is a complicated procedure; the client who may be adjusting normally to a loss and who does not need substantial in-depth therapeutic involvement is as good a case for services as one requiring more therapeutic work. Coordination of services of supportive personnel and professional personnel is a substantial part of the work of the rehabilitation counselor. In many cases, he will have to bring this team together in order that the client can continue to receive effective and necessary rehabilitation services.

The rehabilitation counselor must actively involve himself within the community in order to be fully aware of the many resources which exist that can be of substantial benefit to his clients. Generally, counselors have indicated that so much of their time is taken with counseling and coordination of services that they are unable to put forward enough effort to learn all that the community has to offer. Counselors who utilize community resources effectively are very familiar with the offerings of various agencies and through coordination and cooperation find that their work load is lessened by the support of other social service programs.

The counselor will wish to offer his services to various types of community agencies. For instance, most counselors can give a great deal of useful advice to such programs as the community action and model cities efforts sponsored by the federal government. Agencies and organizations such as family service programs and welfare agencies can be of considerable help in getting needed services for the rehabilitation client. The counselor should take a major responsibility in coordinating efforts of agencies and programs that can help in the rehabilitation of clients, and he should volunteer his time and energies to help strengthen other social service programs.

The rehabilitation counselor must keep in mind that he should be moving the client toward end objectives of independence and successful adjustment on the job. Rehabilitation differs from some other social service professions in the regard that a substantial test of the counselor's work is made at the end of the rehabilitation process. That test consists of the appropriateness of the client's behavior in work situation (Hardy, 1972).

Rehabilitation Counseling with the Blind and Severely Visually Impaired

No special counseling theory need be constructed in order for the rehabilitation counselor to serve blind persons. There is, however, a substantial body of knowledge with which the counselor should be thoroughly familiar. Topics include the etiology of diseases related to blindness, problems in adjustment to visual loss including mobility, social adjustment, occupational advice, and job placement. The counselor serving blind persons has a real responsibility to undertake considerable study in order to acquaint himself with what Father Carroll (1961) has called in the title of his book, *Blindness: What It Is, What It Does, and How to Live With It.*

The rehabilitation counselor serving blind persons has as much or more of a coordinating function as does the counselor in a general agency setting. A counselor concerned with the blind will work closely with the educational services specialist, the social worker, the ophthalmologist, the placement specialist, the rehabilitation teacher, and the mobility instructor who help in the team effort of moving the blind individual toward adjustment to his visual problem and later to adjustment on the job.

Rehabilitation counselors serving the blind, just as counselors working with any other rehabilitation client, must be certain that their clients are without need of further medical or psychological treatment. In this regard, the counselor helping the partially sighted should make certain that no visual aid or professional service can offer additional help to the client. He should be fully aware of the various problems which go hand in hand with a loss of sight. Persons who are experiencing a severe physical inadequacy lose some ability to be independent. They feel socially inadequate and in some cases may have additional problems which at first might not be apparent to the counselor. Advanced age or other physical incapabilities may add to the blind person's adjustment problems.

The client will be very much interested in the prognosis for his future, and the rehabilitation counselor should make sure that valid information is provided. An effective counselor must be ready to help the blind person understand what his opportunities are for education, employment, and social activities. He should also talk with those persons who give information to the blind client, especially professional individuals such as ophthalmologists, to make certain that they have useful information concerning blindness and the services of the state rehabilitation agency.

Bauman and Yoder (1966) have suggested that the rehabilitation counselor must offer:

> a combination of several qualities: (1) his own emotional acceptance of blindness (he must be the first person to whom the client has spoken who did not immediately show great pity and anxiety — a helping new experience for the client); (2) formal or informal instruction in procedures which make it easier to live as a blind person (the home teacher and also some adjustment on prevocational training can help here); (3) realistic planning for the future, including vocational planning if the age and general health of the client make this appropriate. It is true that all of these may be rejected for a time, in which case the counselor must offer (4) understanding, patience, and a gentle persistence which keeps him available until the client and his family are able to reorient themselves to the future instead of clinging to the past.

In counseling with blind persons, the rehabilitation counselor must remember that he is working with individuals who cannot see or whose sight is impaired. The client will differ from fellow blind persons as much as he will differ from sighted persons. Some blind persons are very healthy; others are sickly. Some are well adjusted psychologically; others are poorly adjusted. In many cases, blindness will have caused severe psychological stress which has not been overcome, just as an accident or some other type of traumatic experience may have caused either a sighted or a blind person severe psychological difficulty.

Often, reaction to partial vision causes as much or more frustration and anxiety than reaction to total blindness. One reason for this seems to be that partially sighted persons are unable to function normally and do not want to accept their loss of sight as a reality. They live in a no-man's-world between blindness and sight.

The rehabilitation counselor serving blind and severely visually impaired persons must be even more planful and thoughtful than the counselor who is concerned with individuals who are sighted. Often it will be necessary to anticipate problems which may arise for the blind client. For instance, simply getting to and from the counselor's office may become a very troublesome and embarrassing task. The blind client may be traveling over unfamiliar terrain with or without the help of relatives or friends. The counselor, in many cases, may want to visit initially in the home and later during the relationship invite the client to the rehabilitation agency.

The counselor must be very much aware that this blind client is *tuned in* to auditory clues (*yes*s and *unhum*s may be helpful), since the usual eye contact and other nonverbal communications are not effective with blind persons. For instances, silence over a considerable period of time often takes place in counseling sessions, but when the counselor is working with a blind client, silence may be interpreted at times as disinterest or rejection.

It is respectful and appropriate for the counselor to look directly into the face and eyes of the client just as if the counselee were fully sighted. Blind persons are often aware that sighted persons are not looking at them and they get the impression, which may be true, that the counselor is not listening.

Counselors should be particularly careful about shuffling papers, tapping a pencil on the desk, or making other sounds that are distracting. They should also be aware that many blind persons, especially the congenitally blind, give the counselor little to go by in terms of facial expression. The counselor who is used to reading emotionality in various facial responses may be at a considerable loss with some persons who have been blind for a number of years and who are not nearly as responsive in this respect as sighted people (Jordan, 1962).

A rehabilitation counselor providing professional services to blind persons must avoid fostering unnecessary dependence. Often counselors, unknowingly as well as knowingly, build their own self-esteem by continually allowing clients to rely on them for personal advice and other services. On the other hand, many rehabilitation counselors are afraid to show sufficient interest in the problems of the client because they are concerned about being forced to give a great deal of time and attention to the client. Neither of these extremes will allow the counselor to be effective.

It has been said that the most important variable for helping people which the counselor brings to the counseling relationship is *himself*. The rehabilitation counselor, whether he is working with blind or sighted clients, must make a substantial effort to maintain genuineness, openness, sincerity, honesty, and respect for the client. While techniques and procedures are important in accomplishing goals in counseling sessions, the real key to successful counseling is whether the counselor genuinely cares for the individual. A rehabilitation counselor provides substantial professional and coordinated services from which the client benefits enormously. Most rehabilitation counselors will have certain quotas to meet and the effective counselor, through proper caseload management, will be able to provide quality and quantity services. He will also realize that his coordinative and facilitative function is as important as his counseling function. He must serve clients according to *their needs* and not his own; when this is done, counselees will not claim that his work lacks quality because he will have been much more concerned with them as individuals than with whether or not his services were *professional* in nature.

VOCATIONAL PLACEMENT AND BLINDNESS

There are many commonalities between approaches to the placement of the generally handicapped and those persons who are visually handicapped. Many persons who have visual problems also have a second handicap. One of the purposes of this section is to provide general information which will be useful in vocational placement.

One of the most substantial contributions a rehabilitation counselor can make which affects his client's overall mental and physical adjustment is the placement of the individual on a job that is well suited to his abilities and interests. Vocational placement is underrated by many rehabilitation counselors and others who do not understand the full effects of its outcome. Helping the client find employment is often relegated to scanning newspaper want ads in search of opportunities or responding to a call from an employer who happens to have a job available. Certainly, occupational opportunities can be located through these means; however, the matching of the individual and the job is a complicated process which requires careful study and evaluation through interrelating all casework data on the individual with all information that can be secured relating to job requirements and job settings.

Vocational Placement and Blind Persons

Blindness is a severe disability, and the counselor concerned with the placement of blind persons must be certain that the placement program is carefully planned. No magic is involved in the placement of the blind in competitive employment; however, a great deal of hard work and effective public relations are necessary.

There are many special considerations and much pertinent information with which the placement counselor must be very familiar. For instance, he should have some understanding of the physiological aspects of loss of sight. Such information can be obtained through the study of the medical aspects of blindness. The counselor will need to have answers readily available to many questions concerning the client's adjustment, his ability to communicate with others, to get to his work station, and to get to and from work. The better the counselor understands his client, the more effective he will be in vocational placement. One of the most important concepts for the counselor to remember in working with blind persons is that blind persons are people first and blind second. There are varying levels of potential according to the individual's personality and general intelligence.

A very important aspect of the placement of blind persons concerns getting the client psychologically ready for employment. He must believe in his own ability to do the work which is necessary and he must have confidence in the counselor's judgment concerning the types of jobs he can perform.

Blind workers have proven themselves over the years to be safe, dedicated, loyal, and low in absenteeism (American

Mutual Insurance Alliance). Job opportunities for blind persons cover a very wide range and no list of jobs that blind people can perform is ever appropriate or complete. When he is helping the blind person decide on his vocational future, the counselor should remember that key sources of information for counseling are the client himself and his family. Counselors must move away from stereotyping jobs for blind persons and toward innovative placement. A great deal of information must be acquired about the client through interviews and counseling sessions with him and his family. It can be highly effective in counseling and psychological evaluation of blind persons to ask about the types of job fields they would be most interested in if they were fully sighted. This allows a broad vocational exploration which brings out many possible areas for consideration. Often, jobs in the suggested fields or in closely related ones are feasible.

The counselor concerned with the placement of blind persons will find that many industrial jobs do not require sight. Some of the jobs which do not require sight are the very ones which employers and counselors have thought definitely required sight. Blind persons, according to the legal definition, may have various amounts of vision up to 20/200 in the best eye with best correction or a visual field not exceeding an angle greater than twenty degrees (Jones, 1962). The counselor will have to know his client physically, psychologically, and socially and proceed with the placement plan after all information has been carefully studied and interrelated. Jobs can be evaluated with specific clients in mind or the counselor can approach the evaluation of jobs with various levels of required vision in mind. Again, the key to successful placement is careful planning. The counselor must think of various contingent possibilities. It is most helpful to observe workers performing jobs and to talk with them concerning all aspects of the jobs under observation, including whether they continue to do the job under consideration hour after hour, day after day without modification during all periods and seasons. This approach is often necessary in evaluating the job for a blind worker.

Generally speaking, blind persons continue to need the rehabilitation counselor in a salesmanship capacity. Most blind persons need help in selling their abilities to prospective employers. This is another reason why the work of vocational placement in rehabilitation counseling of the blind persons has great importance.

The remaining sections of this chapter will offer various types of information which will be useful to the rehabilitation counselor serving blind individuals.

A Science of Vocational Behavior

Lofquist and Dawis (1969) discussed a *science of vocational behavior* which they see as essentially vocational psychology. Whether one agrees or not that the science of vocational behavior is actually vocational psychology, the necessity for the full development of vocational behavior study as a science cannot be over stressed. The substantial growth during recent years of interest in the Vocational Evaluation and Work Adjustment Division of the National Rehabilitation Association and the subsequent publication of the *Vocational Evaluation and Work Adjustment Bulletin* have done a great deal to stimulate thinking and research on vocational behavior and practical problems of the individual and groups in the world of work. Certainly, in the future, vocational adjustment studies and work evaluation will take an even more prominent place in the rehabilitation counselor's work and in rehabilitation counselor education within university settings.

Above all, the rehabilitation counselor must be able to understand the *work personality* of his client. The *work personality profile* consists of such factors as vocational and avocational interests; abilities, needs, work habits; psychological maturity; and interaction with on-the-job factors including job hierarchies, communication, and health factors.

The rehabilitation counselor interested in developing expertise in placement should become familiar with available research on work adjustment. Studies done in vocational rehabilitation at the University of Minnesota (Lofquist, 1957) since 1957 offer a great deal of useful information.

Client-Centered Placement

Rehabilitationists have heard much about *client-centered counseling* over the years. Because placement is an important part of the rehabilitation process, counselors should think of *client-centered placement.* Job placement is a major client service which has helped rehabilitation agencies in getting substantial amounts of federal and state funds for program operations. The goal of work is one of the unique characteristics of rehabilitation. The placement of individuals on jobs through which they can find methods to maintain themselves is the concept which has allowed rehabilitation counseling to gain in stature as a social service profession with a substantial contribution to make to the individual and to society. In fact, most laymen would probably say that the location of appropriate jobs for clients is the main function of the rehabilitation counselor. It is interesting that rehabilitation counselors downplay the importance of placement in their jobs when they describe their activities to their friends and colleagues. Counselors might reflect more seriously upon their placement responsibilities if clients were thought of as consumers of their services and were given an opportunity to actually evaluate the jobs which they have obtained with the help of the counselor.

In fact, the use of the phrase *PLACE in employment* is one which misleads the rehabilitation counselor trainee and others concerning the method which should be used. The client and counselor must work together in order for the client to reach a decision concerning the type of job he wishes to have. After this decision is made and the rehabilitation counselor helps the client secure information about various jobs that exist in the geographical area where he wants to be employed, the client himself should take some initiative whenever possible to get employment with the assistance of the counselor. Once a feasible job is located, the client should be given the opportunity to evaluate it as the source of his future livelihood.

Quite often, when considering placement, the counselor is

confronted with the dilemma of determining to whom he owes basic loyalty, the client or the employer; that is, should he be protective of the client when dealing with an employer or protective of the employer. How much of the client's problems and disability should the counselor relate to the employer? Should he obscure the client's disability in discussion with the employer?

If the professional relationship was bilateral and concerned only the client and counselor, the answer to the dilemma would be immediately obvious; however, the relationship is trilateral.

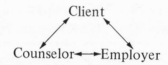

As such, the counselor owes equal professional responsibility to both the client and prospective employer. Therefore, the counselor should communicate with employer in a basic, forthright manner. The counselor is professionally obligated to be honest in his dealings with employer.

If the counselor fails to be completely honest and forthright with the employer, he not only jeopardizes his professional relationship with this employer, thereby obviating any possibility of placing clients in this area in the future, but he also takes a great chance of jeopardizing the client-employer relationship later when the employer becomes more aware of the client's attributes which the counselor chose to hide or misrepresent. Consequently, I feel rather strongly that the counselor should discuss with the client what he is planning to relate to the employer. If the client refuses to allow the counselor to discuss his assets, liabilities, and disability with the employer, the counselor should modify his role in the placement process. His role should be one of providing placement information to the client, but he should not enter actively into the placement process with the client.

There are two limits to this interchange between the counselor and employer relative to the client and they are the following:

1. The counselor and employer should discuss thoroughly those aspects and only those aspects of the client's background which have a direct relation with the job.
2. The counselor should communicate with the employer on a level at which both are comfortable in the exchange of information.

Quite often a counselor approaches a prospective employer regarding a specific client and as the conversation progresses, the counselor finds himself relating information which, while highly pertinent in the rehabilitation process, has little to do with the client as an employee. In each instance in which the counselor makes an employee contact for placement purposes, the counselor should have previously summarized all material in the case folder which is directly related to the client's proficiency in a particular position — both his assets and liabilities. After reviewing this summary, the counselor should refrain from relating any other information he may have derived from counseling sessions, training evaluations, or diagnostic work-ups. A mark of professionalism is the ability to communicate the essential factors relating to the client and still respect the client's fundamental right to confidentiality of case material.

The second limitation to communication between the counselor and employer requires the counselor to assess the sophistication of the employer and to communicate with him on that level. As a general rule, the counselor should avoid using terminology which, though descriptive, is highly laden with emotional connotations. The most effective approach the counselor can take in discussing the client's assets and liabilities is to describe behavior rather than categorizing behavior with diagnostic labels. It is much more effective to relate to an employer that a client experienced learning difficulties in the academic areas rather early and is slow in learning new procedures, is ineffective in dealing with abstract concepts and carrying out complex, oral instructions, and should not be placed in a situation requiring independent judgments in changing conditions but that he is very adept in performing concrete forms of tasks and is capable of making routine, repetitive judgments, than to relate to the employer merely that the client is a mental retardate and assume the employer is sophisticated enough to translate this diagnostic label into behavioristic terms as described above rather than stereotyping the client immediately with a diagnostic label.

Developing an Employment Program

Counselors who are involved with placement should be familiar with information offered in the publication, *Workers Worth Their Hire* (American Mutual Insurance Alliance), which is available through the President's Committee on Employment of the Physically Handicapped. Myths concerning employment of the handicapped are dispelled by information given in this publication. Counselors will find that discussions of the excellent record of handicapped persons in such areas as safety, absenteeism, production, and motivation to work are of considerable help to them in their discussion with employers, union leaders, and work supervisors. The counselor should be certain that he not only talks about these factors with top agency employment officials, but also that he manages, at the appropriate time, to mention these subjects to supervisors within the work area. The degree of acceptance which supervisors give to handicapped clients is often highly influential in not only helping them *get off to a good start* but also in maintaining their work at a level commensurate with the supervisor's expectations.

Some rehabilitation counselors have felt that the counselor should not have a specific client in mind when talking with an employer, but that he should sell the concept of hiring the handicapped to the employer and later get into the work setting in order to locate the types of jobs which would be available to handicapped individuals. This concept can be extremely useful and can help open many doors to blind employees; however, after convincing the employer of the value of hiring blind persons, the counselor often will be asked to refer a prospective employee immediately if a particular opening exists in the work setting. If a counselor is unable to meet this request, his public relations and sales program can be substantially damaged in terms of future placements with the employer.

Each rehabilitation counselor should constantly evaluate his efforts in placement to make certain that he is moving clients toward jobs in line with their overall adjustment and ability. One of the key sources of learning about job opportunities for any client is often the client's past experiences and previous job responsibilities. In many cases, clients will wish to return to the type of employment held prior to the onset of the employment handicap. In fact, many former employers will feel a responsibility for injured employees and wish again to offer them employment after they have received rehabilitation services. The client will offer many insights about himself to the counselor who then has the responsibility to match abilities, needs, and interests of the client with requirements and offerings of the job. One of the primary sources, then, of information about types of employment for the client is the client himself. This information can be gained by a study of his background and from interest inventories and interviews with him and his family.

The counselor will also wish to use the services of the state employment agency which maintains local offices throughout the United States. Many prospective employers inform the employment service of job openings. This agency also offers counseling, placement, and evaluation services for handicapped job applicants. The Vocational Rehabilitation Act, Public Law 89-565, stipulates that the vocational rehabilitation state plan shall "provide for entering into cooperative agreements with the system of public employment offices in the state and the maximum utilization of the job placement and employment counseling services and other services and facilities of such offices."

Questions Counselors Must Be Able to Answer

Of course, many different problem areas can arise when the counselor is discussing hiring handicapped workers with an employer. Questions range from "How will the person get to the place of employment?" to "What will he do in case of fire?" Incidentally, these two questions usually can be answered with the same responses which any employee would give (in the first case, "By bus or car," and in the second, "Get the hell out like everyone else.").

The first basic question which usually arises is that of increased insurance rates if handicapped workers are employed. This is most often an honest employer reaction to the question concerning employment of handicapped workers. Insurance rates would rise if individuals were employed in an agency which tended to have more accidents; however, handicapped workers have been proven to be as safe in the performance of their duties as other workers. In fact, some handicapped persons such as the blind have actually shown better records for safety than nonhandicapped workers. The counselor should have this information readily available and indicate to the prospective employer that indeed, workmen's compensation insurance rates are determined, in part, according to the relative hazards of the work done by the industry in question. Yearly rates also are determined according to the industry's record of accidents and insurance claims. These are good reasons for hiring handicapped workers. If an employer persists in believing that his insurance rates will increase, the counselor should ask him to contact his insurance agent or read again his insurance contract.

A second question which often arises is this: "Why should I hire a handicapped individual when I can employ normal persons whom I can count on for employment without difficulty?"

The counselor will have to answer this question according to his own philosophy and training. Some helpful responses might include the following:

1. Asking why he should not employ individuals whose employment records have been proven and who are well known and highly recommended by rehabilitation employment specialists.

2. Describing the medical, social, and psychiatric evaluations completed on all clients (not being specific or violating confidentiality). In other words, why not hire an individual who comes to the employer in the sense *certified* as ready for em-

ployment?

3. Reminding him that he is actually supporting what he, as a taxpayer, has already invested some money in — an employment program for the handicapped which has proven to be highly successful.

Another question which frequently is raised in employment interviews concerns the firing or dismissal of the employee and the employer's reluctance to treat the rehabilitant in the same manner as he would treat other employees. The counselor again will have to rely on his own resources; however, an analogy may be helpful here: If a salesman were selling refrigerators and the employer bought one which later malfunctioned, the salesman would stand by his product and attempt to get it in good working order. The counselor could briefly discuss follow-up procedures with the employer at this time. He might also indicate that once the handicapped employee has worked for the employer for a time, the employer will feel that he is a fully functioning, well-adjusted employee who should be treated just as all other employees are. The counselor should assure the employer of his confidence in the client.

A fourth question which counselors must be ready to answer concerns architectural barriers and physical limitations of the work setting. Counselors should be frank in their responses to questions concerning limitations of the client and restrictions imposed by the work testing. The counselor should be the first to indicate that certain jobs are infeasible for many of his clients. He should be certain to get across to the employer the fact that he is not going to place a blind person on an unsafe job or on a job which he cannot handle.

A fifth question which often arises concerning employment of the handicapped is that of the *second injury* which might result in total disability and affect the workmen's compensation payments made by the employer. In a vast majority of states and the District of Columbia and Puerto Rico, *second injury* funds or equivalent arrangements have been established. In these localities, the employer is responsible only for the last injury and the employee is compensated for the disability which results from combined injuries.

Some Guidelines and Tools in Locating Employment Opportunities

The following are some suggestions:

1. The counselor should be aware of industrial developments within the area that he serves and in adjacent areas.

2. The three volumes of the *Dictionary of Occupational Titles* (1965) offer a wealth of useful information for rehabilitation counselors. Much emphasis is given to descriptions of physical and personality requirements for various jobs. In addition, these volumes can help expand the counselor's concepts about various types of jobs which are related to the general interest area of the rehabilitation client.

3. Employers with whom former clients have been placed can be important sources of information.

4. Previously rehabilitated clients can offer many sound ideas about existing employment opportunities.

5. Local chambers of commerce usually provide an industrial index which lists types of work available in their communities. Counselors also should coordinate their efforts with those of the state employment service since the mutual sharing of job information can be valuable to both employment services counselors and rehabilitation counselors.

6. When placing persons on jobs in rural areas, the worker should consider enlisting the support of local community leaders such as doctors, city councilmen, postmasters, and religious leaders as well as Rotary, Kiwanis, and other civic groups.

7. If the counselor is interested in assisting individuals in becoming small business managers and operators, he should get in touch with the Small Business Administration office serving his local area.

Professional Placement

In rehabilitation jargon, *professional placement* generally means developing client employment opportunities which require at least a college education. Bauman and Yoder (1962) offer excellent coverage of this area of placement as it pertains to work for the blind. Professional placement is *facilitative* work for the counselor. The counselor can help his client in terms of giving advice and information; however, he must be certain not to take the place of the client in securing actual jobs. The client must be ready to meet with the employer without the counselor in order to discuss his professional qualifications for work. When he has a particular problem, the counselor should be able to assist him with information which could be helpful during the employer interview. For example, he should be coached on how to present himself most favorably. The counselor might help his client develop a resume or portfolio which would outline his training and give examples of any previous work done in the job field in which he wants employment. Other procedures usually followed in placement may or may not be appropriate according to the judgment of the counselor.

A worker in charge of professional placement may want to organize pre-college orientation groups for clients. It will be necessary, also, for the counselor who is dealing with persons in training to inform them about services available while they are in training and away from their home area. If, for instance, clients are attending college, the rehabilitation counselor should help them become acquainted with college counseling center services at the institution they attend (Hardy, 1965).

Effective professional placement requires long-range planning on the part of both counselor and client. Two years before placement (in training cases) is not too early for the client to begin planning with his counselor in order to solve problems related to his securing the type of employment he wants. The counselor will need to prepare by knowing who the prospective employers are and the requirements of the job.

Getting the Client Ready for Employment

Planning for placement does not begin once the client has had vocational training and is ready *skillwise* for employment, but when the counselor first reads the client's rehabilitation referral form. The rehabilitation worker must constantly learn about his client in order to effectively help him secure the type of employment he needs. Jeffrey (1969) has developed a job readiness test which helps in the evaluation of job preparedness of clients. While the total instrument is not applicable to all rehabilitation clients, certain questions are quite helpful with most rehabilitation clients.

Role playing is an excellent method to use in preparing a client for employment interviews. After going through a mock interview which includes a variety of questions, the counselor can give suggestions concerning how the client might improve the impression he makes with the employer. In role playing, it is helpful for the counselor as well as the client to play the role of the employer. Once this is tried, counselors will immediately realize the usefulness of this procedure. The client should realize that getting a job is not an easy task and that he, to the best of his ability, should participate in the job-securing aspects of placement. In some cases, it is an indicator of effective rehabilitation procedures when the client is able to, in fact, *get his own job*, assuming of course that he is ready for employment. The ability with which the client will be able to do this will vary with his motivation and the severity of his social, mental, or physical handicap.

The rehabilitation counselor must stress *training* as a partial answer to many of the problems of the handicapped worker. Overtraining a worker for a job which will affect his personal and family adjustment for many years to come is seldom done. In each case, the counselor must take an individual approach to helping his client. In the case of those who are educationally or socially retarded, various remedial programs may be necessary before actual work training programs can begin. In each case, the counselor must exercise considerable judgment concerning what his client needs in order to be totally ready for employment.

On-the-job training can be a very effective arrangement for client training. In many of these cases, the state rehabilitation agency will make *tuition* payments to the employer-trainer in order that the rehabilitation counselor may get the employer interested in training a client and evaluating his work. It may be necessary for the counselor to help the employer arrange the appropriate payment schedule for the client since he is not a trained employee and would not receive an amount equal to a regularly salaried employee.

Bridges (1946) offered four major factors which are involved in successful employment of handicapped workers. These remain as highly important considerations for the counselor and are listed below:

1. The worker should have the ability to accomplish the task efficiently, i.e. to be able to meet the physical demands of the job.
2. The worker should not be a hazard to himself.
3. The worker must not jeopardize the safety of others.
4. The job should not aggravate the disability or handicap of the worker.

Common Misconceptions about Vocational Placement

Misconceptions about vocational placement are as follows:

1. Because placement occurs toward the end of the rehabilitation process, the counselor's responsibility to the client diminishes.
2. Placement is an activity which requires no counselor training and is a matter of matching an available client with an average job.
3. Client location of his job (*self-placement*) cannot be effective rehabilitation work.
4. When a client is ready for vocational placement, the information in his case folder is no longer of value to his counselor since the client has been, in a sense, readied for employment.
5. Follow-up after placement always can be handled easily by phone or mail communications with the employer or client.
6. Labor market trends and job information and analysis are

the responsibilities of placement specialists and employment service counselors, not of general rehabilitation counselors. 7. An employer will notify the counselor and the rehabilitation agency when he is dissatisfied with a client placement. 8. An employer will automatically call upon the rehabilitation agency to furnish him with additional employees when he needs them.

Rehabilitation counselors should be certain that their clients understand that it is not necessarily bad to be turned down for a job. Counselors should understand that experience has shown that nine or ten employer contacts often must be made before the counselor makes a placement.

Job Analysis

Every rehabilitation counselor should be thoroughly familiar with the techniques of job analysis for use in selective placement. The rehabilitation counselor has to be able to match the prospective worker's social, mental, and physical qualifications with requirements of the job. Factors such as judgment, initiative, alertness, and general health and capability must always be taken into consideration as well as the individual's social and economic background.

Job analysis should answer certain questions concerning the job. *What* does the worker do in terms of physical and mental effort that goes into the work situation? *How* is the work done? In other words, does this job involve the use of equipment, mathematics, or does it require travel? *Why* does the worker perform the job? This component of the job analysis answers the question concerning the overall purpose or the sum total of the task and is the reason for doing the job. The worker also should understand the relationship of his task to other tasks that make up the total job.

Generally, the rehabilitation counselor should attempt to place clients on jobs which they can *handle* and which do not require modification. In some cases, however, minor modifications can be made with little or no reengineering effort. The counselor will have to be careful in suggesting reengineering of a job, since this can be a costly undertaking in many instances. The major objective should be that of helping handicapped workers integrate effectively into the total work force without major modification or change in the work situation.

The following outline can be used in evaluating a job which is to be performed by a handicapped worker:

1. Name used for position surveyed:
   a. D.O.T. title:
   b. Alternate titles:
   c. D.O.T. definitions:
   d. Items worked on in plant surveyed:
2. Usual operator:
   a. Sex:
   b. General characteristics:
3. Physical and psychological demands:
   a. Activities:
   b. Working conditions:
   c. Skill required:
   d. Intelligence:
   e. Temperament:
   f. Other:
4. Description of physical activities:
5. Description of working conditions:
6. Description of hazards:
7. Steps required to accomplish the goal of the work:
   a.
   b.
   c.
   d.
   e.
8. Equipment found in the particular plant surveyed:
   a. Identification:
   b. Set-up and maintenance:
   c. Modification (if required for blind persons):
9. Equipment variations which may be found in other plants:
10. Pre-employment training required:
11. Training procedure:

12. Production:
   a. Full production definition:
   b. Time to reach normal efficiency:
13. Interrelation with preceding and succeeding jobs:

Relating Psychological Data to Job Analysis Information in Vocational Placement

As a first step in getting to know clients well, the counselor should make arrangements to secure appropriate psychological information about them. He should either complete job analyses or use available job evaluation data to make decisions about types of information which will be of value to his clients in the job selection and placement procedure. In many instances, however, the counselor fails to synthesize information obtained from two of his most important sources: the psychological evaluation and the job analysis.

The counselor should take five basic steps, as described by Hardy (1969), in developing a successful procedure for interrelating and using important information. He should do the following:

1. Study the needs of the client and the types of satisfaction meaningful to him.

2. Make certain that valid psychological and job analysis data have been gathered.

3. Review the requirements of the job and evaluate the individual traits needed to meet job requirements.

4. Consider the environmental pressures with which the individual must interact.

5. Discuss the job analysis and psychological evaluation with the client so that he will understand what the work will require of him and what it will offer.

Both client and counselor need to have an understanding of job requirements in order to make realistic decisions. One important move should be structuring a set of goals — a guide to help the client avoid useless foundering that gets him nowhere. What satisfaction is he seeking? What is important to him in the long run and what types of work or work settings will provide these satisfactions? These are questions which the counselor must help the client answer.

Maslow (1954) has suggested a hierarchy of the individual needs which the counselor must understand in order to evaluate a client's psychological status — his satisfactions and frustrations. In the usual order of prepotency these needs are for the following:

1. Physiological satisfaction.
2. Safety.
3. Belongingness and love.
4. Importance, respect, self-esteem, independence.
5. Information.
6. Understanding.
7. Beauty.
8. Self-actualization.

In our society, there is no single situation which is potentially more capable of giving satisfaction at all levels of these needs than a person's work, and it is the responsibility of the counselor to help his counselee plan for future happiness through adjustment on the job.

The worker needs to help his client become fully aware of the social pressures of the job, because these are as important to the individual as the actual job pressures. A client's ability to adapt to the social interactions of the work environment will directly affect his job performance.

The counselor always must ask himself what the requirements of the job are. This question can be answered superficially or in considerable detail. A lay job analyst can give superficial requirements, but the responsibility for an in-depth job description belongs to the expert — the counselor who will often have to give direct advice to the client.

Effective placement requires effective planning. Planning cannot be really useful unless appropriate information has been obtained, interrelated, and skillfully utilized so that the client and the counselor have a clear understanding of possible problems and possible solutions.

Follow-up After Placement

A rehabilitation counselor often is tempted to consider his job completed when the client is placed on a job which appears suitable for him; however, the phase of rehabilitation which begins immediately after the person has been placed in employment is one of the most complex. Follow-up involves the counselor's ability to work as a middleman between employer and client in order to help the client solve problems related to his handicap which may arise after being hired. The counselor must be diplomatic and resourceful in maintaining the employer's confidence in his client's ability to do the job. At the same time, he must let the client know that he has full faith in him. The counselor, however, must somehow evaluate how his client is performing on the job and make certain that he is available to help if problems arise which the client cannot solve.

In addition to the worker's service to the client during follow-up, this period can offer real public relations opportunities for the counselor, especially when the employer notes the interest with which the counselor *follows* his client. The frequency of follow-up varies according to the counselor's judgment of the client's job ability and adjustment.

Agency regulations usually require that a final follow-up be done after thirty days in order to make certain that placement is successful before a *case* can be closed as rehabilitated. Counselors should also consider follow-up periods of sixty to eighty days after placement. Again, this helps reassure the client of the interest of the agency and the counselor in his success and can be of value to the counselor in further developing employment opportunities for handicapped persons.

In follow-up after professional placement, however, the counselor must increase the sixty to ninety day period which is usually adequate in the placement of clients in nonprofessional jobs. A longer period will be necessary and this period will vary with job complications and severity of the client's handicap. Bauman and Yoder (1962) have recommended six months to a year for follow-up in most cases where blind persons have been placed in professional work.

Counselors will probably wish to schedule specific days for follow-up in the field. Generally, the period of follow-up is a time when the counselor sees the efforts of the entire rehabilitation process coming to fruition. If the job has been well analyzed and the client well evaluated and placed, follow-up will be a pleasurable experience for the counselor.

Summary

The counselor's responsibility in vocational placement must not be underrated. The decisions made at this stage in the rehabilitation process not only affect the client's immediate feelings of satisfaction and achievement but also, of course, his long-term physical and mental health. The counselor has a real responsibility to *ready* the client for employment by giving him the type of information that he needs about the job and about holding employment once it is achieved. Placement should be *client-centered* with strong emphasis given to the client's opinions about work and how it will affect him and his family. Counselors must be ready to answer the questions that employers will ask about hiring handicapped persons and about the rehabilitation program. Vocational placement is high level public relations work.

The counselor must be knowledgeable about job analysis and must interrelate all medical, psychological, and social data with job analysis information in order to be successful in client-centered placement. Once placement has been achieved, the counselor must follow-up the client in order to make certain that he is doing well on the job. The client should have an opportunity to evaluate his job and also the efforts of his counselor in helping him decide on and obtain the job. Effective placement requires effective planning, and counselors must constantly evaluate their knowledge of the world of work and their ability to interrelate information in order to assure real placement success.

References

American Mutual Insurance Alliance: *Workers Worth Their Hire.* Chicago.

American Psychiatric Association: *Diagnostic and Statistical Manual of Mental Disorders.* Washington, D.C., American Psychiatric Association, 1965.

Bauman, Mary K. and Yoder, Norman M.: *Adjustment to Blindness — Re-Viewed.* Springfield, Thomas, 1966.

Bauman, Mary K. and Yoder, Norman M.: *Placing the Blind and Visually Handicapped in Professional Occupations.* HEW, Office of Vocational Rehabilitation, Washington, D.C., U.S. Govt Print Office, 1962.

Bridges, C. C.: *Job Placement of the Physically Handicapped.* New York, McGraw, 1946.

Carroll, Thomas J.: *Blindness: What It Is, What It Does, and How to Live With It.* Boston, Little, 1961.

Department of Veterans Benefits, Veterans Administration: *They Return to Work.* Washington, D.C., U.S. Govt Print Office, 1963.

English, H. B. and English, A. C.: *A Comprehensive Dictionary of Psychological and Psychoanalytical Terms.* New York, McKay, 1966.

Gustard, J. W.: The definition of counseling. In Berdie, R. F.: *Roles and Relationship in Counseling.* Minneapolis, U of Minn, 1953.

Hardy, Richard E.: Counseling physically handicapped college students. *New Outlook for Blind,* 59:5:182-183, 1965.

Hardy, Richard E.: Relating psychological data to job analysis information in vocational counseling. *New Outlook for Blind,* 63:7:202-204, 1969.

Hardy, Richard E.: Vocational placement. In Cull, John G. and Hardy, Richard E.: *Vocational Rehabilitation: Profession and Progress.* Springfield, Thomas, 1972.

International Society for Welfare of Cripples: *Selective Placement of the Handicapped.* New York, 1955.

Jeffrey, David L: Pertinent points on placement. *Clearing House,* Oklahoma State University, November 1969.

Jones, J. W.: Problems in defining and classifying blindness. *New Outlook for Blind,* 56:4:115-121, 1962.

Jordan, John E.: Counseling the blind. *Personnel and Guidance Journal,* 39:3:10-214, 1962.

Lofquist, L. H. and Dawis, R. V.: *Adjustment to Work — A Psychological View of Man's Problems in Work-Oriented Society.* New York, Appleton, July 1967.

McGowan, J. F. and Porter, T. L.: *An Introduction to the Vocational Rehabilitation Process.* HEW, Rehabilitation Services Administration, Washington, D.C., U.S. Govt Print Office, July 1967.

McNamee, H. T. and Jeffrey, R. P.: *Service to the Handicapped 1960.*

Phoenix, Arizona State Employment Service, 1960.

Maslow, A. H.: A theory of human motivation. *Psychological Review, 50*:370-396, 1954.

Morgan, Clayton A.: Personality of counseling. In American Association of Workers for the Blind: *Blindness.* Washington, D.C., AAWB, 1969.

Office of Vocational Rehabilitation: *Training Personnel for the State Vocational Rehabilitation Programs — A Guide for Administrators.* Washington, D.C., U.S. Govt Print Office, 1957.

Sinick, D.: *Placement Training Handbook.* Office of Vocational Rehabilitation, Washington, D.C., U.S. Govt Print Office, 1962.

Stalmaker, W. O., Wright, K. C., and Johnston, L. T.: *Small Business Enterprises in Vocational Rehabilitation.* HEW, Vocational Rehabilitation Administration, Rehabilitation Services Series No. 63-47, Washington, D.C., U.S. Govt Print Office, 1963.

Thomason, B. and Barrett, A.: *The Placement Process in Vocational Rehabilitation Counseling,* HEW, Office of Vocational Rehabilitation, GTP Bull. No. 2, Rehabilitation Services Series No. 545, Washington, D.C., U.S. Govt Print Office, 1960.

Truax, Charles B. and Carkhuff, Robert R.: *Toward Effective Counseling and Psychotherapy: Training and Practice.* Chicago, Aldine, 1967.

United States Employment Service: *Dictionary of Occupational Titles.* Washington, D.C., U.S. Govt Print Office, 1965.

United States Employment Service: *Selected Placement for the Handicapped* (rev. ed.). Washington, D.C., U.S. Govt Print Office, 1945.

Weiss, D. J., Dawis, R. V., Lofquist, L. H., and England, G. W.: *Minnesota Studies in Vocational Rehabilitation.* Minneapolis, University of Minnesota, Industrial Relations Center. (Series published since 1954.)

CHAPTER 12

CONSIDERATIONS IN GRADUATE REHABILITATION COUNSELOR EDUCATION

A. Beatrix Cobb and John G. Cull

REHABILITATION is an interdisciplinarian process which focuses on the individual. We call it a client-centered approach. It is one in which the client is a party to the process and not merely something which is acted upon. The rehabilitation counselor is the model rehabilitation generalist and he is called on to perform an extraordinarily varied range of functions. The counselor must be familiar with the medical aspect of disability. He must be able to integrate and evaluate psychological information. He must understand what work means and be able to develop custom job opportunities and also avenues for self-employment. He must be able to counsel clients to help them with personal problems. He must be a community organizer and a public relations specialist, able to educate the community about rehabilitation and its services. He must be familiar with the contributions of related disciplines such as medicine and, in the case of worker's for the blind, specifically ophthalmology. He must be familiar with other areas such as speech therapy, psychology, occupational and physical therapy, and the many allied health professions. He must be able to serve as the focal agent of all their services. He must understand the functions of sheltered workshops, as well as other types of rehabilitation facilities, and assess their appropriateness for his particular client.

This need for a broad spectrum of skills is reflected in our expectation that counselors serving in the public and private rehabilitation agencies have completed graduate training. This wide scope of required knowledge and practice also is used in defining new patterns of personnel organizations in the delivery of services.

Rehabilitation counseling requires all the ingredients usually accepted as being necessary and required for effective counselor/client relationships. However, much of rehabilitation counseling consists of advice giving and coordination of services to the client. In a sense "rehabilitation counseling" can be considered a misnomer when the term is applied across the board. A substantial number of clients need significant advice and information concerning social and rehabilitation services from which they can profit. When the counselee needs advice and information, the rehabilitation counselor must be able to recognize and meet this need in a professionally acceptable manner. There also will be many instances in which the client and counselor must enter into a number of counseling sessions in depth. The counselor must make the judgment concerning what patterns of help may be needed for the client to solve his particular problems. Rehabilitation counselors need appropriate training to enable them to decide whether or not they are qualified to do the kind of counseling which is necessary.

Many counselors fall into the trap of wanting to play the role of "junior therapist" and involve high percentages of their clients in in-depth counseling sessions. This is particularly true of the graduates of many rehabilitation counselor training programs. Some counselors attempt to justify low agency production with statements which reveal a confusion between the terms "depth" and "quality," a feeling one cannot ensure without the other. In truth, quality counseling and good results can be a product of efficient coordination of needed services (without deep personal involvement) and, on the other hand, there is not proof that in-depth counseling in every case ensures success. Dependency, after all, is a two-way street. In a client, it is understandable — but in a counselor, it borders upon the unacceptable. There is much talk of quality services and in-depth counseling which require considerable time. The rehabilitation counselor who is an effective manager of his caseload can "rehabilitate" the number of persons required by his agency administrator and, while doing so, provide the amount and quality of counseling services needed by his clients.

Rehabilitation work requires a broad definition of counseling which includes the offering of some, and coordination of other, professional services to clients. Generally, agency administrators — especially those trained in counseling — do not accept the explanation of "the time required for quality services" as a rationalization for a low client rehabilitation rate. An agency administrator or supervisor knows that some cases require much involved counseling and that these cases, in many instances, are the most difficult ones. They are time consuming and they can test the fiber of the rehabilitation counselor. Untrained counselors generally cannot handle such cases without help from someone who has had a more advanced orientation to counseling. However, counselors who play the role of junior therapist, trying to become deeply involved with all their clients (whether or not this type of service is called for), will be ineffective and probably will not remain long in rehabilitation work.

The rehabilitation counselor will find his coordinating and facilitating role highly rewarding when it is done well and results in the delivery of needed services to the client. One of the greatest satisfactions that the counselor can have is the assurance that he knows when certain types of services are required and whether these should be more therapeutically oriented or oriented more toward advice-giving, providing information, and coordinating community resources and professional services.

Rehabilitation counselors should not rank order their clients in a psychological need hierarchy which places the individual with severe psychological problems at the top of his list for services. Certainly those persons should be served immediately upon the counselor's realization that severe psychological problems exist. They should be referred to the appropriate psychologists or psychiatrist if problems are so severe the counselor cannot handle them alone, or they should be served by rehabilitation counselors who are competent in providing the type of services required. The point to be made here is that the rehabilitation process is a complicated procedure; the client who may be adjusting normally to a loss and who does not need substantial, in-depth psychotherapeutic involvement is as good a case for services as one requiring more psychotherapeutic work. Coordination of services of supportive personnel and professional personnel is a substantial part of the work of the rehabilitation counselor. In many cases he will have to bring his team together so the client can contribute to receive effective and necessary rehabilitation services.

The rehabilitation counselor must involve himself actively with the community in order to be fully aware of the many resources which exist that can be of substantial benefit to his clients. Generally, counselors have indicated that so much of their time is taken with counseling and coordination of services that they are unable to put forward enough effort to learn all that the community has to offer. Counselors who utilize community resources effectively are very familiar with the offerings of various agencies and professional members of the community, and through coordination and cooperation find that their work load is lessened by the support of other social service programs.

The rehabilitation counselor must keep in mind that he should be moving the client toward the ultimate objectives of independence and successful adjustment on the job. Rehabilitation differs from other social service professions in that a substantial test of the counselor's work is made at the end of the rehabilitation process. This test consists of the appropriateness of the client's behavior in a work situation.

From the beginning, the training of rehabilitation counselors has been a controversial subject. Primarily the debate seems to be rooted in the unresolved problem of rehabilitation counselor roles and functions. Two points of view were set forth in the early days of the profession. Many saw the role as one of a coordinator of services. Others thought the functions described that of a counselor. If the rehabilitation worker was to be a coordinator, certain relevant *training* would be indicated. On the other hand, if the rehabilitation worker was to be a counselor, professional *education* would be required. The operational consensus seems to be that the graduate curriculum should be multidisciplinary in nature with emphasis on developing skills to meet needs which are peculiar to the handicapped.

From the behavioral and social sciences, such subjects as psychology, sociology, anthropology, and economics seemed relevant. In the field of education, areas of special and vocational education appeared pertinent. From health services, medicine, nursing, physical and occupational therapy, and speech and hearing therapy all seemed applicable. The focus on the individual client was borrowed from psychology and medicine. From social work came the emphasis on the importance of family and community group membership. Vocational evaluation was adapted from the fields of vocational counseling and industrial psychology. From vocational education was derived training and placement skills. All of this was then to be superimposed on and mediated through specific knowledge and concern for physical, mental, emotional, and social disability and the impact of the resulting handicap on human behavior and function.

After the consensus of what constitutes a rehabilitation counselor was developed, educators set about describing the training required for the rehabilitation counselor. Generally it has been accepted that the core areas of training include course work in the areas of principles, methods, and techniques of rehabilitation counseling; psychological tests and measurements; psychological and medical aspects of disability; theories and techniques of individual and group counseling; techniques of vocational placement; occupational information; and community services and resources. Course work in this broad area of rehabilitation counseling is accomplished on the graduate level. Many colleges and universities provide this training in departments of education, psychology, sociology, or health related professions. A few have separate departments of rehabilitation counseling.

The counselor training program at the Virginia Commonwealth University is one of the outstanding programs in the United States. The educational formats leading to a master's degree in rehabilitation counseling are varied at Virginia Commonwealth University. An individual may follow the traditional graduate school pathway in which manner he may pursue a degree requiring two years of graduate work including an internship. There are several other educational approaches provided by the Department of Rehabilitation Counseling at Virginia Commonwealth University. Some of these include the work-study program, the Regional Counselor Training Program, and the evening college program, all of which are designed to facilitate the professional practitioner in achieving the graduate degree in rehabilitation counseling. Each of these approaches require forty-seven semester hours of graduate work and, through several different approaches, a substantial amount of clinical experience with disabled individuals.

In summary, the role of graduate training in rehabilitation is to prepare the counselor to undertake the following:

1. To understand disabilities and the vocational implications of disabilities.

2. To counsel with the client toward better adjustment.

3. To utilize and coordinate effecitvely existing medical, paramedical, educational, and community resources in a manner which facilitates the adjustment of the disabled client.

4. To facilitate vocational adjustment through counseling and placement activities.

CHAPTER 13

EVALUATING THE REHABILITATION PATIENT THROUGH PSYCHOLOGICAL AND OTHER DIAGNOSTIC PROCEDURES

MARY K. BAUMAN

WE all evaluate people — people we know well, people we meet casually, people we pass on the street. Indeed, evaluation is so natural a mental function that it is difficult not to do it.

At the very least, we react with evaluative attitudes to the appearance, the manner, and the speech of others, and we are likely to be especially conscious of this kind of quick and perhaps superficial evaluation in the case of an individual we have just met. Given more time in a structured relationship, we evaluate on the more sound basis of observed behavior. Is he punctual, is he cooperative, does he bring to our common concerns any initiative or originality?

Many of us also evaluate on the basis of the individual's history, either as he himself recounts it or as we hear it from others. Has he succeeded in ventures he tried, is he liked by others, has he carried significant responsibilities? A few of us may be in positions where we evaluate on the basis of formal records. In an educational setting we may evaluate on the basis of previous academic records, in a hospital we carefully study previous health records, in some settings evaluation may be influenced by employment records, police records, etc.

Thus evaluation among laymen may be based on any combination of immediate impressions, observed behavior, reported past history, and various kinds of routine records.

Professional Approaches to Evaluation

Professionals in the field of evaluation try to refine all of

164

these lay means of evaluation into more exact measures; they try to reduce the effects of chance. Professionals may structure observations so that all trained observers would pretty much agree in their evaluation of a particular individual. They may weight certain data in an individual's history so that it has more accurate predictive value for a given situation, such as success in college or in a job. Finally, they may present specific tasks in specific ways (tests) in order to get measures upon which there can be no real disagreement — although there may still be disagreement about the predictive value of that measure in relation to school, job, or other kinds of success.

The layman tends to evaluate on the basis of his own experience; when that experience is limited in amount or narrow in nature, his evaluation is likely to be biased. To overcome that, professionals share information, widening the experience of each one to the experience of all. When we have a large enough group of experiences on a sufficiently formal method of evaluation, we call that group of experiences norms. Norms are the most scientifically defensible and the most easily expressed sharing of experience.

Unfortunately, not all kinds of evaluation can readily be put into normative form; this is particularly true of observation as differentiated from specific measurement. Even when the measurement is specific and norms are available, the interpretation of those norms and the suggesting of a sound plan for the individual's future may require a great deal of knowledge of a highly professional nature. It is not too difficult to use tests which result in IQ, interest, and personality scores; what may be difficult is interpreting those scores against the medical, educational, and behavioral background of a specific individual and guiding him to a life plan in which he can be successful and happy.

We can develop dependable norms only when we are exact about what we are counting, so a test is a standard material — verbal or concrete — used in a standard way, yielding some result (number of correct responses, speed of completing a task, number of parts assembled within a time limit, etc.) which can be counted in a standard way and compared with similar results from a standard group — a defined, homogeneous group.

There are many tests for sighted persons, many excellent norms based on large, well-defined populations. Some of these tests have been studied over many years and with large groups of people, especially in relation to measured success in school, college, industry, and certain of the professions. Psychologists of rather limited experience can often use such tests with their sighted clients and, by wise interpretation of the norms which are provided with the test, a rather good career plan might be developed.

Evaluation and Blindness

However, the evaluation of blind people is far less simple for a variety of reasons.

Often it is impossible to use standard test material which was developed for sighted people. Many efforts have been made to adapt tests which have known success with the sighted, but almost invariably the adapted test adds new elements which we did not plan to measure and which may totally confound the norms. For example, Kohs developed a test based on the copying of designs by combining red and white blocks in certain patterns. This test has been so well accepted by psychologists that it is used by itself and as part of several very widely used general mental measures, such as the various forms of the Wechsler tests. Naturally, people have tried to adapt the Kohs test to tactual form so that it could be used with blind persons (Shurrager, 1961; Suinn and Dauterman, 1966) and it is easy enough to make blocks which differ in texture instead of in color. In many ways this adaptation has been successful but there is no doubt that a new element, the requirement for tactual discrimination, has been built into these blocks and for some blind clients tactual discrimination is so poor that the test ceases to be a measure of mental ability only — for a few with extreme discrimination problems, it is frustrating and emotionally upsetting.

In other cases, it may be possible to use standard material but not in a standard way. For example, tests of English, history, or a foreign language might be used without any content change with blind students. However, in most cases the printed test for sighted students would have a time limit; to use the same test for a blind student requires either that it be read to him or that it be put into braille and in either case the time limit of the ink print test must be discarded. Both reading aloud and reading braille are much slower processes than visual reading of ink print by a good student. If we discard the time limits we must also pretty much discard the norms as exact comparisons.

Our description of a test emphasized that the score of the individual must be compared with the scores of a normative group which had considerable homogeneity. In many cases, even when we can use standard test materials in a standard way with the blind client, his life experience is so different from that of the members of the normative group that interpretation is difficult. His schooling may have been interrupted by health and visual problems, he may not have received full opportunity to participate in school and other life experiences, he may have been overprotected or rejected in family and peer relationships, and he has obviously totally lacked some experiences if he was blind from birth. How can we correctly predict the future for him on the basis of norms developed on sighted people with very different life experience?

A natural response to this might be to develop tests especially for blind people and some of this has been done very effectively. The process is a lengthy one, however, because it is difficult to reach large numbers of blind people to test them for the purpose of developing good norms and blind people do not form a homogeneous group. For example, the age at which vision was lost affects whether the blind person can possibly have certain concepts, such as the concept of color. Differences among blind people may also result from differences in kinds of education, in amount and kind of help from agencies, and in the attitudes of family and friends around them, to name only a few of the life influences which may have significant impact.

Despite the need to be aware of, and indeed to beware of, so many factors, the psychologist experienced in evaluation of blind clients can make a considerable contribution to the rehabilitation plan.

Psychological Tests Used with Blind Persons

In evaluation of blind clients, the most widely used and most reliable tests are verbal measures of mental ability, chiefly some form of the Wechsler Scales (Bauman, 1968). These tests were developed for the total population but since they are always administered individually by simple oral questioning they can be used without adaptation for blind clients. Their scores have been related to school and job success and to many aspects of psychosocial adjustment. They can be interpreted for the blind client almost exactly as they are for the sighted person.

The Wechsler scales (WAIS, WISC, WB II) all have performance sections which must be replaced in the case of blind clients by one or more of the performance tests developed for this purpose. Of these, the one most nearly paralleling the WAIS is the Haptic Intelligence Scale (Shurrager, 1961; Shurrager and Shurrager, 1964) which reproduces in three-dimensional form some of the WAIS Performance Scale items and which provides norms on a blind population patterned on the normative population for the WAIS. However, the HIS does have the disadvantages of lacking norms on partially seeing clients, serves only clients sixteen years of age and over, and is quite time consuming to administer.

A performance test which does have norms for the partially seeing and which is somewhat easier to administer is the Stanford Kohs Block Design Test (Suinn and Dauterman, 1966). The blocks have marked contrast between white and black, smooth and rough sides. With as many as sixteen such blocks the client is asked to copy a series of patterns of increasing complexity and providing a wide range in scores. To most people, the task is inherently interesting and highly motivating; but for a few, the fact that the entire test is built around one kind of mental activity may be a disadvantage. Again, unfortunately, norms do not reach below age sixteen.

At younger age levels and for persons of extremely limited ability, a variety of formboards may be used based more on the psychologist's experience with such tasks than on formal norms for blind people. One formboard which shows great flexibility is the Non-language Learning Test (Bauman, 1947; Bauman and Hayes, 1951). Here the basic measurement is that of learning — learning as a result of initial problem solving from which the client may profit to varying degrees, learning from careful instruction by the examiner, and learning from repetition. By varying the initial presentation, the task can be adapted to amount of vision, general mental level, and, to some degree, to the age of the client. These variations make it possible to use the task with persons who are totally blind and with persons with considerable useful vision; it is also possible to make it difficult enough to challenge the capable adult yet it is not without diagnostic value for some preschool children.

Indeed, since the chief purpose for using any of these materials is to predict learning ability with concrete tasks, the experienced psychologist may use other familiar test materials to sample learning. For example, dexterity tests, especially the Minnesota Rate of Manipulation, the Penn Bi-Manual Worksample, and the Small Parts Dexterity Test (Bauman, 1968), provide learning situations in which the client may be observed especially with reference to his ability to follow instructions, maintain his orientation in the work space, and manage changes in the hand used for different parts of the tasks. Of course dexterity tests were designed chiefly to measure speed and coordination on simple manual tasks, the factory kind of job. Their scores relate to the speed with which the task is completed. The experienced psychologist may, however, get much additional information by carefully noting all facets of the client's behavior during the learning period on each test and by observing motivation, attitude, work habits, duration of attention, etc. during the actual performance of these demanding but quite repetitive assignments.

Several standard achievement tests have been put into braille and large print form by the American Printing House for the Blind, a rather complex process in which individual test items are carefully studied, time limits are changed, and much research assures the applicability of the norms provided with the regular print edition of the tests. Thus the academic progress of visually handicapped children can be monitored.

Special aptitude tests may often be used by simply reading them to the blind person although it is necessary to present multiple-choice items with great care. One of the most widely used aptitude tests, the Scholastic Aptitude Test (SAT) has been adapted to braille and tape form by its originators, Educational Testing Service of Princeton, New Jersey.

Some of the well-known personality and interest inventories have been used with blind clients quite successfully and Bauman has developed both personality and interest inventories specifically for blind adolescents and adults (Bauman, Platt and Strauss, 1963; Bauman, 1968; Bauman, 1973). Presentation of such questionnaires by means of tape recordings assures the visually handicapped client of privacy and probably maximizes frankness in responding. Projective personality tests have also been developed (Braverman and Chevigny, 1952; Palacios, 1964) and while these should be given far more careful study and perhaps refinement, they offer useful material to the psychologist already skilled in the interpretation of projectives.

Thus there is available a fairly complete battery of tests for basic diagnosis and for educational and career planning for the visually handicapped child and adult. In most cases the test materials are relatively new and there is less reported research upon their use and long-term followup than is true for similar materials for the sighted, but when carefully interpreted they have considerable value.

Importance of History and Observations

All counselors should use observed behavior and the history of the counselors as verification of test results but this is especially important in working with the blind person.

Good communication between physician and counselor is vital since the career plan should certainly include consideration of present and probably future general health and specific eye conditions. It is extremely helpful if the physician will make himself available for consultation, at least by telephone, when any unusual health condition is present.

Careful analysis of the educational history is also necessary since breaks in the typical educational sequence frequently occur. Variations in quality of or actual gaps in academic preparation can result from the child's absence due to illness, accident, or surgery, or as a result of transfers between day and residential schools, or from lack of appropriate resource room or itinerant teacher support during much of his school life. Since schools are disinclined to penalize blind children for such factors, the child may graduate from high school with acceptable grades but some serious deficits in preparation. The rehabilitation counselor must find some way to correct these deficits before going on with a career plan which depends upon that foundation.

Interpretation of the results of personality and perhaps even interest inventories requires some understanding of family and other attitudes and influences, and the weighing of as many parts of the blind person's life experience as can readily be reached in an interview of normal length. We cannot emphasize too much the importance of such influences in the shaping of the self-concept, motivation, and goals of a visually handicapped person.

In the course of a day of testing simple observation will tell much about the individual's dependency versus initiative and independence, his interest and enthusiasm versus possible depression and withdrawal, his planfulness and drive toward achievement versus lack of any sense of trying for speed or caring about accuracy. The testing situation should also provide some opportunities for observing social behavior, orientation and mobility, capacity to express himself clearly, and of course such characteristics as neatness, cleanliness, and appropriateness of dress. Many of these characteristics are subject to change with training and counseling; negative observations certainly do not close the door to rehabilitation but, rather, they show where rehabilitation must begin.

More Extended Observation

For many people, rehabilitation begins with quite extended periods of observation along with teaching; the observation indicates where the teaching should begin and constantly reflects the changes in the individual which result from teaching. Often it is when we try to change people through some type of teaching and/or counseling that we gain our best understanding of them.

The rehabilitation teacher (formerly known as the home teacher) offers a combination of counseling and teaching especially directed toward independence in daily living and in managing a household. Teaching often includes braille and other communication skills, crafts and recreation, and some beginnings of orientation and mobility. Frequently the rehabilitation teacher is a blind person who can, in addition, offer the model of his own independence as an encouragement to the homebound client.

For many people it is more effective, however, to get out of the home and to learn all of the above independence and communication skills in a rehabilitation center where learning occurs throughout the waking hours. Here training can be far more intensive than any offered in the home, opportunities to use the training are constantly provided, and successful performance on the part of the client is quickly reinforced. In addition, the rehabilitation center can usually offer more kinds of training than can be taken into the home, including development of listening skills, improvement of coordination and physical endurance, skills of group living, and perhaps even prevocational skills. Physical therapy and psychotherapy may be included as needed.

Because the rehabilitation center works with the client over a much longer period of time than does the psychologist in his office, a prolonged kind of testing and observation becomes possible. Many centers have formalized this into what are called worksamples. Some centers prefer worksamples which are actually small parts of jobs imported from local industry; it is hoped that clients who achieve success on such worksamples may be ready for placement on real jobs within those local plants. Other centers have developed joblike segments of activity such as sorting, packing, assembling, checking, etc. Most of these are simpler than the real job would be but by careful observation and timing over a moderately long period, such as a half day, success on the complete job can be predicted.

In the rehabilitation center, intensive mobility instruction almost invariably takes much of the trainee's time. When only orientation and mobility training is needed, it may be provided in the home neighborhood. In any case, mobility instruction includes skills in finding one's way toward more and more distant and difficult goals, usually by cane travel. Where appropriate, the trainee is also taught use of public vehicles such as bus, subway, train, etc. For some, use of a guide dog is the preferred mode of travel; here again intensive training of dog and master together is a necessity. The close relationship between the mobility instructor and the blind client often makes that instructor an important influence toward independence in ways not directly related to mobility, something of a counselor, and certainly an individual who can contribute major insights to the rehabilitation evaluation team.

For young people, educators are inevitably evaluators and not merely in academic matters. Their contribution is so well known that it seems necessary to comment only upon special variations such as the summer programs offered by some states. These programs simulate college experience with dormitory living, attending classes, taking notes, using the library, taking tests, and writing papers. One might call this a kind of halfway house between high school and college where it is possible to learn how nearly the individual is ready for the combined freedom and responsibility of college and at the same time provide training to make him ready.

A somewhat similar tryout for youth who are not college bound may be provided by work-study programs. These schedule students for perhaps a half day of regular school and half day on a real job, preferably outside the school. The young person learns what is expected by an employer — improved work habits, promptness, accountability, and the satisfaction of a job well done. Again the program is at once a means of evaluation and a vehicle for teaching skills and attitudes.

For the adult who does not seem ready for competitive employment, placement in a sheltered workshop may provide a gradual development of skills and good work habits. In the workshop the individual is encouraged to do a real job as quickly and effectively as possible but he is not penalized for failures such as might cost him his job in industry. Observation, evaluation, training, and counseling combine to bring him to his maximum potential as a producer before he tries employment under a less understanding supervisor in a factory or office.

Conclusion

Here, with a brevity which may be supplemented by other publications (Bauman, 1958, 1966, 1968; Lowenfeld, 1973; MacFarland, 1973; Curtis, 1972; Wisland, 1974), we have delineated the most frequent procedures for evaluating the visually handicapped and totally blind youth and adult. Obviously, many of these procedures are used with people in the general population and with other segments of the rehabilitation population. Many are adapted, a few are specific to problems of blindness.

This chapter is intended especially to leave two thoughts in the mind of the reader: (1) There are immense variations among blind people. They vary in all the ways in which other people vary, plus the very complex pattern of potential differences which result from their visual conditions and the psychosocial effects of those conditions. (2) Despite inadequacies of testing instruments; evaluation, counseling, and rehabilitation planning are not only possible but well-established professional offerings. All that is needed is to bring the patient and the rehabilitation process together. In this few can play a more important role than the eye physician.

Bibliography

Bauman, Mary K.: Report on a non-language learning test. AAWB,

Proceedings, 1947, pp. 99-101.

Bauman, Mary K.: *Manual of Norms for Tests Used in Counseling Blind Persons*. New York, Am Foun Blind, 1958.

Bauman, Mary K.: *Tests Used in the Psychological Evaluation of Blind and Visually Handicapped Persons*. Washington, D.C., AAWB, 1968.

Bauman, Mary K.: An interest inventory for the visually handicapped. *Education of the Visually Handicapped*, 5:78-83, 1973.

Bauman, Mary K.: Psychological and educational assessment. In Lowenfeld, Berthold (Ed.): *The Visually Handicapped Child in School*. New York, John Day, 1973.

Bauman, Mary K. and Hayes, Samuel P.: *A Manual for the Psychological Examination of the Adult Blind*. New York, Psych Corp. HarBraceJ, 1951.

Bauman, Mary K., Platt, Henry, and Strauss, Susan: A measure of personality for blind adolescents. *International Journal for the Education of the Blind*, *13*:7-12, 1963.

Bauman, Mary K. and Yoder, Norman M.: *Adjustment to Blindness — Re-Viewed*. Springfield, Thomas, 1966.

Braverman, Sydell and Chevigny, Hector: *The Auditory Projective Test*. New York, Am Foun Blind, 1952.

Curtis, W. Scott: *The Development and Application of Intelligence Tests for the Blind: A Research Utilization Conference*. Athens, Georgia, University of Georgia, 1972.

Lowenfeld, Berthold: *The Visually Handicapped Child in School*. New York, John Day, 1973.

MacFarland, Douglas C.: The blind and the visually impaired. In Garrett, James F. and Levine, Edna S. (Eds.): *Rehabilitation Practices with the Physically Disabled*. New York, Columbia U Pr, 1973, pp. 431-460.

Palacios, May H.: *The Sound Test: An Auditory Technique*. Marion, Indiana, Author, 1964.

Shurrager, Harriett C.: *A Haptic Intelligence Scale for Adult Blind*. Chicago, Illinois Institute of Technology, 1961.

Suinn, Richard M. and Dauterman, William L.: *Manual for the Stanford-Kohs Block Design Test for the Blind*. Stanford, California, Stanford University School of Medicine, 1966.

Wisland, Milton V. (Ed.): *Psychoeducational Diagnosis of Exceptional Children*. Springfield, Thomas, 1974.

CHAPTER 14

RIGHTS OF BLIND CONSUMERS OF MEDICAL AND REHABILITATION SERVICES

John G. Cull and Kathy F. Levinson

In questioning the adequacy of service programs with which rehabilitation agencies meet the needs and rights of consumers, we feel there is a discrepancy between consumer oriented attitudes and the actual delivery of services to the consumer.

Traditionally, rehabilitation service programs have prided themselves on being client oriented, or at least since the passage of the Barden-LaFollette Act of 1943. However, our experience leads us to believe that more physicians and rehabilitation practitioners need to have the basic rights of blind clients — within the medical and vocational rehabilitation process — identified, clarified, and incorporated into their delivery of services. The purpose of this paper is to discuss some of the basic rights of blind clients in the rehabilitation process.

Basically consumers of services have two types of rights. These rights may be divided into categories according to the recourse the consumer has when his rights are violated. The consumer has legal rights and professional rights. With the first type the individual whose rights are violated has recourse through the legal system. With the second type the individual is protected by the professional ethics of the provider of services and the ethical stance of his profession. Historically, consumers of services have felt sufficiently protected by the professional ethics of providers of services. However, in the last decade there has been a decided shift in this perception of the adequacy of the protection of consumer rights. The result has been a correspondent increase in consumers seeking recourse to violations of

176

their rights. One may observe this shift by noting the increased incidence of legal suits being brought against providers of services. Perhaps the greatest shift we have observed is in the area of medical and health care services. All of us are acutely aware of the magnitude of malpractice suits brought against physicians, clinics, hospitals, and others in the health care delivery systems. Recently rehabilitation practitioners have become more concerned relative to their liability in the delivery of rehabilitation services. This concern is reflected in the increasing number of rehabilitation practitioners, including rehabilitation counselors, who are purchasing malpractice insurance.

Perhaps the most basic right of the visually impaired individual is the right to receive vocational rehabilitation services. Prior to the 1965 amendments to the Vocational Rehabilitation Act, the provision of vocational rehabilitation services was a privilege which might or might not have been provided. Subsequent to the 1965 amendments, the provision of services is a basic right of the visually impaired individual, providing of course the disabled individual meets the three criteria of eligibility. This change in concept and client rights resulted from the provision of an appeals process to challenge decisions made by the rehabilitation counselor with which the visually impaired individual disagreed. With the advent of the appeals process, the applicant for rehabilitation services gained a legal right to access to services.

The client has a right to have explained to him, in terms he can understand, the goals, functions, procedures, and operations of the agency. He has a right to know and understand from whom he is receiving services and the ramifications of his accepting services. As a part of this right the client may accept or reject services from the rehabilitation agency without being subjected to coercion or having prejudicial evaluations of him being made by the rehabilitation counselor or the rehabilitation agency. This is a right, we feel, all of us demand when we ourselves are consumers of services; therefore, it is only fair that we provide the same consumer options we demand. This right also applies to the patient who is to receive medical services from the ophthalmologist. The blind person who is coming to the ophthalmologist for medical services should be made aware in detail of the medical process including diagnosis, treatment, prognosis, and medical follow-up. In short, the patient should be an equal partner in the medical and vocational rehabilitation process and not be considered merely a passive recipient of these services.

Related to this is the client's right to be informed of their rights in the rehabilitation process. As such it is incumbent upon a professional representative of the agency to discuss these rights with the client at the beginning of the rehabilitation process. This presents an interesting dilemma to the rehabilitation counselor. He should discuss these rights with the client, yet few rehabilitation counselors are aware of these rights. Therefore, the clients' rights often are violated because of this lack of understanding.

Throughout the rehabilitation process, but especially during the initial phases, the client has the right to receive appropriate referral and advocacy services in instances when his particular needs cannot be met by the rehabilitation agency. This is a professional right as opposed to a legal right, but we feel it is just as binding. Referral and advocacy, part of the counseling obligations of the counselor, require a relatively comprehensive understanding of community resources and particularly other social services agencies, including their eligibility criteria, the specific services they offer, and the circumstances under which the services may be provided.

Referral and advocacy means the client may justifiably expect the rehabilitation counselor not only to identify probable service agencies which might meet the disabled individual's needs, but also expect the rehabilitation counselor to refer the client to those agencies and, if indicated, to actually become an advocate in assisting him to receive the needed services. We feel much of the frustration and disenchantment many clients feel, as a result of being shuttled from one agency to another, comes from the lack of proper referral and advocacy services.

The client has a right to be apprised of the appeals process of the state rehabilitation agency. He has the right to develop an understanding of this process and how to initiate the process. This means the rehabilitation counselor is professionally obligated to ensure the client's understanding of the appeals mechanism. Even though a rehabilitation counselor may fulfill his legal obligation by sandwiching in a brief mention of appeals between several other topics or activities in the initial phase of the rehabilitation process, it by no means indicates he has fulfilled his professional obligation in an adequate or acceptable manner. To fulfill this professional counseling obligation the rehabilitation counselor must ensure that the client understands the nature and procedures of appeals, the means by which he initiates an appeal, and that one may initiate an appeal without jeopardizing the opportunity to receive services.

The client has the right to an impartial, thorough, and professional evaluation to determine his eligibility or ineligibility for services regardless of the particular circumstances. This includes the right to an adequate medical diagnostic work-up which is definitive in its indication of the presence or absence of a medically determinable disability. This right also includes the client's right to receive a thorough evaluation of his rehabilitation potential.

If after receiving a thorough, impartial, professional evaluation the disabled individual is found to be ineligible to receive services he has three distinct rights — the right to be informed of the finding of his ineligibility, the right to reapply for services, and the right to a periodic review and reassessment of his ineligibility. Often counselors feel that the applicant who is found to be ineligible does not have the right to reapply for services unless there has been a significant change in his situation. This is not the case. The disabled individual has the right to apply for services at any time he chooses to do so. There are no limitations we know of which constrict the individual's options to apply to the agency for services.

At times, rehabilitation counselors violate the consumer's rights by failing to notify him of his ineligibility due to an adverse finding on the part of the rehabilitation counselor. The applicant not only should be notified of his ineligibility but the rehabilitation counselor should share with the applicant the rationale for this determination. We feel that better explanations of the rationale behind a finding of ineligibility will result in fewer reapplications.

As a result of recent federal legislation (Public Law 93-112) the rehabilitation counselor is now legally mandated to periodically review and reassess determination of ineligibility. This reassessment must be made at least annually and the consumer must be afforded a clear opportunity for full consultation in the reconsideration of the ineligibility decision.

The visually impaired client has the basic right to be a full partner in the planning of services which are to be received to assist him in achieving vocational stability. This means the partnership role should be identifiable to the extent that the rehabilitation counselor can demonstrate, if called upon to do so, the impact the client had in determining the vocational objective, the array of services to be provided, the intermediate and long-range behavioral objectives, and the strategy or order of provision of services. Rehabilitation administrators and professional practitioners assumed for years that the client was a full partner in this planning; however, upon reviews of actual practice across the country it was found that this basic consumer right was being violated so prevalently that the 1973 Rehabilitation Act mandated the Individualized Written Rehabilitation Program (IWRP) to ensure client participation in planning for services. The client should have the freedom to reject a particular constellation of services without fear of the rehabilitation counselor reacting in a prejudicial manner to the detriment of the client. For example, if the client is unduly fearful and apprehensive regarding surgery, he should have the right to reject surgery as an option to increase his level of physical functioning to ensure vocational stability. If this occurs, it is incumbent upon the rehabilitation counselor to counsel (*not coerce*) the client relative to the implications of refusing surgery. If the client remains adamant, then it is the professional responsibility of the rehabilitation counselor to plan around the visual disability as it exists. A complete violation of the client's rights as well as professional ethics occurs when the rehabilitation counselor threatens a client in this set of circumstances with the withholding of services if he does not acquiesce to surgery.

Related to the above right is the consumer's right to have a major role in the selection of the providers of services. We feel that unless the rehabilitation counselor has a compelling reason which indicates he override the client's selection of a particular provider of service, the rehabilitation counselor should recognize the client's preferences. If the rehabilitation counselor does have this compelling reason which justifies overriding the client, the rehabilitation counselor should deal with the conflict between himself and the client through a counseling approach rather than by an authoritarian fiat. In the past, when the provision of services was based on privilege rather than rights, we could more easily and safely direct the client through this authoritarian frame of reference; however, with the advent of the appeals process counselors are finding more demands are being made on their counseling skills.

The client has a right to expect a periodic review and modification, if indicated, of intermediate and long-range vocational and behavioral objectives as outlined in the Individualized Written Rehabilitation Program. Neither the rehabilitation process nor the IWRP is a self-sustaining or self-perpetuating structure. That is, even though they are progressing smoothly both the rehabilitation counselor and client should continue to evaluate both the adequacy of movement toward the goals of the rehabilitation process and the appropriateness of the goals. If the movement toward the goals exceeds the expectations of the rehabilitation counselor and client, the client rightfully should expect either the goals will be raised or the time spent receiving services will be decreased. If, on the other hand, the client is achieving the intermediate behavioral objectives at a significantly slower pace than anticipated, the client has a right to expect appropriate modifications be made in the strategy of provision of rehabilitation services. The implication of this right is that the client justifiably should expect a continuum of involvement with the rehabilitation counselor — not, as occurs in many cases, to be set adrift after the development of the IWRP.

The client has the right to share in all employment decisions and activities made in his behalf. He has a right to expect more than merely being offered a job. He should be involved in evaluating the various placement alternatives to assist in screening some in and screening some out, rather than being offered a specific placement option as a *fait accompli*. The client should be totally privy to the details and results of interactions between the rehabilitation counselor and the prospective employer if the client is not present during the interaction. Related to this right is the consumer's right to expect an active effective follow-up after placement to facilitate his development on the job. And the disabled individual has the right to expect this follow-up to continue until vocational stability has indeed been accomplished. The implication of this right is that closure is the result of a joint decision on the part of the client and the rehabilitation counselor. In many instances the client is unaware of when the case is closed. This is a violation of the client's consumer rights, also it is a violation of good professional practice in rehabilitation.

Just as the visually disabled individual has the legal right to receive rehabilitation services, he has a corresponding right to receive post-employment services to continue to ensure his vocational stability and productive viability. While the client has no legal rights to receive specific rehabilitation services or post-employment services, he does have a right to receive those services he and his rehabilitation counselor feel will be necessary to accomplish the goals of the rehabilitation process. Therefore, denying a rehabilitated client access to post-employment services is equivalent to denying rehabilitation services to an applicant who has met the three criteria of eligibility.

Several rights the consumer has pervade the entire rehabilitation process — from initial interview through closure and into the provision of post-employment services. One of these rights is the right of access to material directly related to the client which the rehabilitation counselor has gathered from secondary sources. This includes medical evaluation data, psychological data, vocational evaluative data, medical treatment data, and training evaluations. The client also has a right of access to data in the case folder which has been generated by the agency, such as continuing contact reports. In complying with these rights the rehabilitation counselor needs to exercise wise and mature professional judgment, for one of the most basic principles of counseling is: communicate with the counselee on the level at which he is equipped to understand. Therefore, the rehabilitation counselor should share information with the client in such a manner as to ensure the information will not be damaging to the client and in such a manner that the client will understand what is being shared.

During all phases of the process the client has the right to both prompt decision making on the part of the rehabilitation counselor and the agency as well as prompt services. The counselor must realize that most clients are eager to return to work and in many cases, are prepared to move more rapidly than the bureaucratic structure of the agency can accommodate them. The client has every right to expect the counselor to be his advocate in facilitating his moving through the process and into vocational stability as rapidly as possible rather than the rehabilitation counselor becoming a part of the bureaucratic structure which impedes the rehabilitation process. This implies that the rehabilitation counselor must make decisions on a timely basis rather than delaying them. He also must facilitate the initiation of services just as rapidly.

The client and the disabled in our communities now may justifiably expect to have a dynamic role in making state rehabilitation agency policy and effecting changes in existing policy. This consumer right was given to consumers as a result of the Rehabilitation Act of 1973 which stipulates the views of recipients of rehabilitation services or their representatives shall be considered in general policy development or policy implementation. This provision has spurred the development of consumer advisory boards and committees whose responsibility is to provide input on consumer views and values to the state agency.

Lastly, the client has the right to expect the highest quality professional attention available from the rehabilitation counselor. The rehabilitation counselor must take part in programs of self-development to continue upgrading his skills to even better serve the disabled who, in many cases, so desperately need his professional skills. Also, the rehabilitation counselor should not sacrifice the needs of the client for the benefit of any other party involved in the rehabilitation process. This includes the employer, the state rehabilitation agency, or even the counselor himself.

In summarizing the consumer's rights in the rehabilitation process, we find ourselves reiterating concepts and phrases which have become worn, trite, or hackneyed. Perhaps it all boils down to the Golden Rule — clients in the rehabilitation process should be served by the rehabilitation counselor in the manner in which the rehabilitation counselor would like to be served were he to become a client. While this philosophy lacks freshness it does have powerful implications — it is the basis of client centered counseling; violation of it causes the legislative mandate of IWRP. Violation of the above philosophical approach to rehabilitation has resulted in the need to initiate client assistance projects around the country and has caused a marked increase in the incidence of litigation.

CHAPTER 15

REALISTIC NEEDS OF THE BLINDED INDIVIDUAL

Louis H. Rives, Jr

I THINK that at the outset I should point out that my assessment of the needs of blind people is no doubt colored by my own experience. I speak from the perspective of a blind person who lost his sight at the age of two because of retinal blastoma, who attended a school for the blind for three years, who completed his elementary and secondary education in regular classes in a public school system, who completed college and law school, and who has had by the standards of our time a successful career in public administration — a large part of which has been concerned directly with services to blind people. During the time when I was attending school and making decisions about my career, there was not much formalized assistance for blind persons available but I did receive a great amount of help from family, teachers, friends, and finally from an employer who was willing to take a chance on hiring a blind attorney. This help has been augmented along the way by a lot of luck and considerable persistence.

In this chapter, I shall try to base my remarks on observations and analysis rather than on my personal experience with the hope that they will be objective. In the broadest sense, the needs of a blind person are exactly the same needs that he would have if he could see. These needs differ just as people differ. Each blind person has — in relation to his own personality, self-concept, and intellectual capacity — basic needs for economic security, self expression, social intercourse, success, competition, love, privacy, recreation, approval of his peers, and personal dignity. Just as for people who can see, all of these needs are seldom fully met. We cannot expect that they will be fully met for blind people; but the true job of rehabilitation, in which the ophthalmologist plays a vital role, is to do everything possible to remove the barriers which the fact of blindness places between the individual and the fulfillment of these basic needs.

Other chapters of this book will deal in depth with the services and techniques which are available to assist blind people. I want to concentrate here on the needs of the blind person from the point of view of the ophthalmologist and on the need for the blind person to learn to manage his handicap from the point of view of the rehabilitation agency.

The patient who is about to lose his sight has certain specific needs which can be met only by the ophthalmologist. These include the following: (1) The provision of the best medical and surgical skills to prevent blindness or restore sight. Fortunately, this need is met for most persons. (2) When, despite the use of the ophthalmologist's best skills, it becomes clear that the patient is going to be blind the patient has a need to know this and the ophthalmologist has a responsibility to tell him. Though it may seem cruel to make a patient face the stark fact that he is blind and that there is no hope for recovery, it is in reality much more cruel to give false hope or to temporize. It has been demonstrated time and time again that because of the tremendous fear of blindness, individuals will cling to the slightest hope that they will see again and will not accept the fact that they are going blind. Until the individual accepts this fact, he cannot begin the slow and difficult process of learning to cope with blindness. (3) At the same time that the ophthalmologist brings his patient face to face with the harsh fact of blindness, he should also let his patient know that there is help available to assist him in the difficult process of adjustment. The physician should know what resources are available in the community including low vision aid clinics for patients with some residual vision and should make sure that the patient is put in touch with these resources. (4) If the patient's eye condition is inheritable, the physician should make sure that the patient understands this fact and what its implications will be. (5) Finally, the ophthalmologist can provide a major service to his blind patient by demonstrating his continuing interest in him by following up to see that the rehabilitation and other agencies are serving his patient just as he would if the patient were referred for auxiliary medical services.

In summary, the blind patient needs from the ophthalmologist medical skill, truth, help, hope, and continuing interest. If he receives less, the ophthalmologist has not met his patient's needs.

The rehabilitation agency in the broadest sense has the overall responsibility for assisting the blind person in meeting those needs which will enable him to function at his maximal potential despite his handicap. They include a thorough medical, vocational, psychological, and social diagnosis and a plan of rehabilitation services based on these diagnoses and the delivery of the requisite medical, social, training, counseling, and placement services needed to achieve the goal of the rehabilitation plan. Each of these areas is being dealt with by other authors in this book. In addition to these services, and perhaps in the long run of even more importance, is the need of the blind person to learn to manage and accommodate to the constraints which blindness puts upon him. Some of the elements, such as those following, involved in the personal management of blindness can be taught by competent instructors and learned with varying degrees of effectiveness by blind persons who are motivated to strive to achieve independence: (1) Mobility and orientation skills which enable a blind person to move from one place to another with a maximum of efficiency, comfort, and safety and with a minimum of emotional stress. The degree of mobility which can be achieved, of course, varies with each individual's capacity. (2) Skills in the activity of daily living which include such elements as the development of table etiquette acceptable to the persons with whom he will be associating, personal grooming, and the awareness of appropriate clothing and color coordination. (3) The development of some system for the keeping of his personal records either in braille or recorded form.

Each of these elements is also being presented in depth by other authors in this book. In addition, however, there are certain intangible factors relating to the management of blindness which cannot be taught but which must be acquired through counseling, observation, experience, and introspection. These include the following: (1) A realistic acceptance of the limitations which blindness imposes, coupled with an equally realistic awareness of the myriad activities in which a blind person can engage. (2) An acceptance of the fact that there are certain activities in which sighted assistance will be required. A blind person must learn to identify those situations in which he needs assistance, to seek that assistance with a minimum of inconvenience to his sighted helpers and gracefully to get rid of the sighted help when it is not needed or when it becomes stifling. (3) The capacity to convey to the general public what it is that they can expect or not expect of blind people so that eventually each blind person can be judged on his own merit rather than being viewed with wonder or pity or both.

I have highlighted some basic needs of blind people as they must be met by the ophthalmologist and by the rehabilitation complex. To the extent that each of these key professions discharges its responsibilities, blind people will have the opportunity, though not the guarantee, of a full and rewarding life. To the extent that they do not meet these responsibilities, blind people will be short-changed.

CHAPTER 16

ATTITUDINAL AND COUNSELING CONSIDERATIONS IN THE REHABILITATION OF THE BLIND

RICHARD S. LUCK AND JOHN G. CULL

Introduction

PROFESSIONAL rehabilitation workers with the blind require a great deal of expertise in and knowledge of a vast array of technical, medical, and professional information. Since blindness is one of the most, if not the most, feared of all disabilities by the lay public, rehabilitation workers need also to be acutely aware of negative attitudes that impinge upon the rights of the blind individual. These attitudes affect the blind person's psychological adjustment to the disability and the blind person's ability to form a positive counseling relationship. Special attention in this chapter is focused upon these attitudinal considerations, especially the impact of blindness upon the individual's psychological adjustment to disability and the ability to enter into a counseling relationship. Emphasis also is placed upon several counseling techniques that do not work with the blind and some positive counselor attitudes which may help the blind client in his adjustment to disability.

Cull (1975) has written extensively about the psychological adjustment to blindness. He has illustrated an adjustment curve that the newly blinded person goes through. This process has been illustrated in light of the ego defense mechanisms that the person employs. The thesis is that the greater the quantity and richer the quality of the use of these ego defense mechanisms, the more rapid and positive will be the person's adjustment to disability. There are several implications for the professional

189

rehabilitation worker with the blind that are important to enumerate in light of this proposition.

First of all, it is imperative to view blindness from a functional point of view rather than an anatomical one. This is important for both the blind client and the professional worker. The crucial concept is to capitalize on the functional abilities the person has left and not on the functional limitations. The focus must be squarely placed on ability, not disability, and on the person as a total individual.

Secondly, it is imperative that the blind have information which is factual, concise, and clear. It is highly desirable that the person or persons who provide counseling for the blind be sure that the client's perception of blindness is correct and that every detail regarding the cause is completely understood. The responsibility of the counselor is to help provide this information in the form which the client can best understand. The provision of the information must be tailored to fit the client's needs and to facilitate his understanding on a timely basis. The counselor must guard against providing both too little and too much information. The task is to provide only that which the client is ready for and needs at the time he needs it.

Thirdly, the client may need to be helped in exploring his feelings regarding the manner in which he is currently being treated by family and friends. The psychological adjustment curve developed by Cull (1972) not only holds true for the blinded client but aids in understanding the psychological reactions of his family and friends as well. These significant others may be adjusting to the client's blindness also, and they may treat him differently for a while. In some cases the blind person may adjust to the disability at a more rapid pace than his significant others. The influence of family and friends can either help or hinder the client in his adjustment depending upon the client's understanding of the emotions involved and the attitudes that these people hold towards him. These attitudes will dictate to a large degree the treatment he receives from these other persons. The blind person also has a great deal of influence over the attitudes that these other people have towards him. He can very subtly encourage these people either to treat him as an invalid who needs constant care and sympathy or as an independent person who may require some assistance from time to time.

Next it is important for rehabilitation professionals to avoid the trap of thinking that the degree of blindness is directly correlated with the degree of psychological impact. Blindness is a highly individualized phenomenon and is dependent upon a variety of factors. Each of these individual factors must be examined and considered on an individual basis; there is no pat adjustment formula to blindness. Furthermore, it is important that professionals be warm and empathic toward the client and accepting of the client and his situation. The development of a positive attitude toward the client is a must. The professional will want to strive to be pragmatic in guidance and planning and supportive and steadfast in counseling.

The professional also will do well to avoid thinking that because the client has accepted his blindness he has adjusted to it in a positive manner. Acceptance must come first; however, it may be based on faulty data or negative attitudes. It is wise for the professional worker to examine thoroughly the acceptance. The possibility exists that the professional worker may have to counsel with the newly blinded client to "reaccept" disability before the client can be helped to adjust to it in a positive manner.

Finally, and of primary importance, is the concept that an individual's adjustment to his disability is dependent upon the attitudes he had prior to the onset of the disability. If his attitudes towards the blind in general were quite negative and strong, he naturally will have a greater adjustment problem than an individual with a positive attitude towards the blind or blindness. A part of this attitude formation prior to blindness is dependent upon the experiences the client had with other blind individuals and the stereotypes he developed. This idea will be discussed in more detail later in this chapter.

Attitudes Defined

The term attitude has been mentioned several times and before continuing perhaps it is necessary to examine the construct called attitude. An attitude is a psychological construct, that is, it cannot be observed directly (Wallace, 1972). It cannot be seen, touched, smelled, or heard; it is intangible. However, the manifestation of an attitude can be observed in human behavior. Attitudes influence behavior in either a positive or a negative manner. They affect the way an individual acts or reacts. People may respond with either aversion or enthusiasm, not only towards activities but also towards social groups, institutions, individuals, and many other factors in the person's environment.

An attitude then is a feeling state, an affective phenomenon. It is a feeling of favorableness or unfavorableness towards some activity, individual, group, institution, or proposition. Attitudes have been further defined as the stands a person takes and cherishes about objects, issues, persons, groups, institutions, etc. (Sherif, 1965). These stands usually are well entrenched and extremely resistant to change. The stand a person takes most likely involves a commitment; the person commits himself to a certain position which subsequently influences his behavior. Attitudes are intricately interwoven into a person's value system and are the basis upon which many sacred personal beliefs are founded.

An attitude is a preconditioned mind set that is learned due to experience and observation of a role model such as parents, close friends, admired leaders, or public heroes. Everyone holds attitudes of some sort or another and all human behavior is greatly influenced by them.

In addition, attitudes are formed socially and they are selective. They are learned from one or a combination of the following sources and many are formed in early childhood. These sources include the following (Sartain, 1962):

1. Specific experiences and observations.
2. Communications from others (especially parents, teachers, and close friends).
3. Imitation of models (a very important source of learning which has tremendous implications for rehabilitation professionals).

4. Institutional factors such as the military, the church, and government.

These sources and others transmit attitudes which are either positive or negative. Attitudes are never neutral; either an attitude exists or it does not. If it does exist, it is either favorable or unfavorable.

The emphasis in this chapter is upon negative attitudes, their identification, influence, and modification. Negative attitudes towards blindness must be modified or changed to more positive attitudes if they are to help rather than hinder the psychological adjustment to blindness and societal acceptance of the blind.

Sources of Attitudes Towards Blindness

There are perhaps more references in the Bible towards blindness than any other single disability. Obermann (1965) listed many of these, among which was Leviticus 21:18-21 which set certain standards for priests. "For whatsoever man he be that hath a blemish, he shall not approach 'to offer the bread of his God.' A blind man, or a lame, . . . or dwarfed or that hath a blemish in his eye. . . . He hath a blemish, he shall not come nigh to offer the bread of his God." Compassion is urged in other passages, for example, "Cursed be he that maketh the blind to wander out of the way" (Deut. 27:18). Disability, sickness, and disease were, and unfortunately still are, interpreted by many as an expression of displeasure of the Lord. Religious attitudes are especially difficult to change because religious teachings and beliefs form the core of many people's value system.

The agricultural and industrial society in the United States perceived blindness to be the most debilitating disability. A society which highly valued productivity could not imagine how a person could work with his hands and be productive if he could not see with his eyes. In light of this, it is interesting to consider the political pressure that brought about the tax law that enables a person to take an extra exemption on the federal income tax return for blindness. This is the only disability for which this is allowed. The blind and the elderly are the only two categories that are permitted to take an extra exemption, the reason being that the productivity of these groups is considered negligible in an agricultural and industrial society.

Blindness is one of the few if not the only disability with a legally specified definition. Blindness is legally defined for an individual from a critical point in the range of visual acuity as one who has not more than 20/200 of visual acuity in the better eye with corrective lenses. This definition is also referred to as industrial blindness. The popular lay definition of a blind person, however, is simply "one who cannot see."

The vocational rehabilitation act of 1973 specifically designates blindness as a severe disability. Many agencies for the blind distinguish between blindness as a severe disability and other visual disabilities by the person's inability to obtain a driver's permit.

The ancient occupation for the blind has been begging (unable to see — unable to work). However, during the early Middle Ages the blind bard became an occupational type. Some learned to play musical instruments as well as sing and recite poetry (Obermann, 1965). This is still a noble occupation for many blind persons today. One has only to recall the blind guitar player downtown on the street corner or better yet, think of some of the great popular musicians like Ray Charles, Stevie Wonder, and Jose Feliciano.

Separation of the blind into asylums, schools, workshops, and occupations has been practiced for centuries. Many blind persons have been isolated in a type of closed society. As a result, blindness has come to be regarded (attitudinally) as a mysterious and awesome thing. Limited expectations, limited performance, and limited opportunity have been the result of the practice of isolating the blind. The pygmalion effect has been perpetuated by society upon the blind. The pygmalion effect greatly paraphrased is "what you expect is what you get." Society traditionally has expected little from, and provided even less opportunity for, the blind. There are exceptions to this of course, like the American Association of Workers for the Blind and other groups. However, the blind have had an extremely difficult time in securing competitive employment. For example, how many blind public school teachers are there for sighted children? Even at this writing the authors know of only one who secured employment as a public school teacher, and only then after suing the board of education in her state.

A story by Ernest Hemingway perhaps is illustrative of the attitudes held towards blindness as one of the most debilitating disabilities. The story illustrates that blindness is one of the worst things that could happen to someone, or if one were to inflict a disability upon another that blindness would be one of the most extreme ways. Hemingway, in *Death in The Afternoon* tells the story of two gypsy children who followed a bull which had killed their older brother. They followed this bull hoping to see him meet with his death; however, this never happened and the bull became very old and was sold to a man who was going to slaughter and butcher the animal for meat. The gypsy children sought the bull out and inquired of the man that owned him if they might unleash their vengeance upon him before he was butchered. Having gotten the owner's permission, the two children set about to do injury to the bull. They began first by blinding the bull; secondly they castrated the bull; thirdly they killed the bull. After having killed the bull they stopped in the streets, roasted his testicles, ate them, and then went their way. The most vengeful acts the gypsy children could perform were first to blind, second to castrate, and third to kill.

There is an indication that many Spanish-speaking persons associate blindness in the male with sexual impotence. One of the authors having worked along the Mexican border of the United States has noticed that many young adventitiously blinded Mexican and Mexican-American males also suffer from sexual impotence.

Negative Attitudes Towards Blindness

Attitudes are either singular or interrelated and linked together. The following five attitudes are presented as if there is a pattern or interrelationship. An individual can harbor any of these attitudes singularly or in any combination; however, it is often the case that these five form a pattern or constellation of attitudes towards the blind.

Fear

The first and perhaps most formidable of the attitudes under consideration is fear. The individual is afraid of all connotations of blindness, all the dark, evil, ignorance, and mystery involved in shadow and gloom. Fear is an emotional or vague feeling, a state of extreme discomfort and insecurity. It may be irrational and unconscious. It is the feeling that someone or something is out to get you. The fear under consideration is based upon irrational or false beliefs. Why would anyone be fearful of a blind person? Because he can not see? It just does not make any sense; it is an unfounded fear. For some strange reason, blindness is equated with evil and people should fear evil things because they will do you harm.

Blindness is to be feared, just like any other disability, but in a positive, rational way. Since we are positively fearful of becoming blinded, we use good sense and take precautions to protect our sight. For example, fear prompts us to wear safety glasses when operating dangerous machinery.

Fear in a negative sense, however, causes us to be afraid of the suspected effects of blindness, the irrational effects such as the loss of reality contact (being cut off and isolated from others), the loss of work (financial insecurity), loss of our normal mode of adjustment to living (immobility and dependence), and above all mutilation and the unknown. We know these irrational fears often become reality; however, we also know that this need not happen.

Revulsion

The second attitude which is important for our consideration is revulsion. Fear leads to revulsion. Because of the fear we experience, based on faulty logic, we attempt to obliterate from existence, or at least from consciousness, those things we fear. This results in the denial or avoidance of the things we fear. We run away or stay away from the things we fear, or we keep those things we fear in a safe place like in an asylum, prison, workshop, school, or home for the blind.

Pity

Pity comes about next as a compensation for revulsion. Fear and revulsion are not socially acceptable so we attempt to cover them up by pitying the object we fear and wish to eliminate. Pity is useful in that it helps separate the object of pity from ourselves. We become apart from the poor blind beggar on the corner. Pity is selfish, it helps us to cope with our fears. It also fosters dependency for the person pitied, not independence because we need him to handle our fear and our guilt feelings. Pity is coupled with sympathy. Sympathy is self-serving, it is the "there but for the grace of God go I" attitude. It helps us find security and solace in the fact that "I'm glad that never happened to me," "I sure am lucky."

Prejudice

These three — fear, revulsion, and pity — lead to prejudice. Prejudice is a global attitude which is unfavorable or negative. It is emotionally resistant to change and actively resistant to all evidence that would unseat it. Usually it is learned as a young child, primarily from parents. Children tend to perpetuate the prejudices of their parents and therefore it is basically a deep-seated emotional belief that spans generations. Some of the factors associated with prejudice are the following:

1. Socioeconomic status seems to be related to prejudice. Certain socioeconomic groups tend to hold the same prejudices.

2. Individual personality — due to unconscious anxieties and hostilities learned or transmitted from significant others. Frequently prejudice is a projection based upon anxieties

and reinforcing experiences.

3. Prejudice usually comes in clusters and involves dogmatic thinking. In this fashion, prejudice becomes bigotry. For example, in consideration of disability, "Not only do I not like blind people, I don't like deaf-mutes, arthritics, epileptics, crazy people, or any other cripple." This attitude is perhaps best expressed popularly as "Archie Bunkerism."

Stereotyping

Finally, prejudice leads to stereotyping, the "you've seen one — you've seen them all" attitude. "I've seen the dirty blind begger down on the corner who chews tobacco, smells foul, plays the guitar, and sleeps in the gutter. Therefore, all blind people chew tobacco, smell foul, sleep in the gutter, play the guitar, and, most importantly, must be beggers to earn a living." Stereotypic thinking in the aforementioned manner is indicative of common attitudes towards blindness.

False Generalization

These five attitudes, either on an individual basis or linked together in a constellation, lead us to make false generalizations such as some of the following regarding blindness:

"It's amazing how they can tell color just by feeling it."
"They are all so carefree and happy."
"Never saw one who couldn't play a musical instrument."
"If you work for the blind you must know the sign language." (This is a typical confusion of blindness with other disabilities.)
"Ask him if he wants sugar in his coffee." (This is indicative of the tendency to feel the need to speak to a blind person through a third person.)

Two Principles (Hypotheses)

In light of all this one may wonder what is the point. The

point precisely is that both blind people and professional workers with the blind are not protected from holding these same attitudes. In many instances we are not even conscious of the fact that we hold these attitudes. Imagine the detriment to the blind person's psychological adjustment to blindness if he held these attitudes prior to becoming blind. The fact that he was blinded and now is blind will not automatically change his negative attitude. He will not only continue to hold those same negative attitudes about blind people in general, but he will now hold these attitudes about himself. He will begin to include himself in the very group about which he has negative attitudes. We have labeled this phenomenon as *the principle of self-inclusion.*

The second principle is called *the principle of general inclusion.* Not only will the blind person feel this way about himself, but he will also believe that everyone else feels the same way (that he himself feels) about this group and him as a member of the group. The important thing is that the blind person may accept his disability based upon these two principles which is, of course, a negative acceptance to blindness that will lead to a negative adjustment to blindness or at least prevent a positive adjustment.

Modification of Negative Attitudes Towards Blindness

There are several ways that negative attitudes can be modified. It is generally accepted that the most effective way is through intergroup contact or interaction. When prejudiced people are brought into direct contact with minority group members and share experiences with them, attitudes often undergo a gradual but deep change. The principle upon which this is based is that familiarity with the attitude stimulus diminishes the unconscious fear of the unknown, since such fears often are unfounded and based on ignorance.

A second way is through direct educational programs. Familiarization with accurate information can contribute directly to amelioration of the cultural atmosphere in which undesirable attitudes breed.

A third way is through changing the attitudinal environment of the prejudiced individual. People desire to accept the views of those with whom they identify. A person seeing others around him changing their attitudes is relieved of vague fears and can change with them. People who carry prestige in the eyes of the conformer can effect a change, particularly if their statements are backed by action and not contradicted by other people of higher prestige. Professional rehabilitation workers are such people. This is extremely important in rehabilitation workers' contacts with clients and others. They are a model whether they wish to be or not. If the professional rehabilitation worker accepts the blind client it makes it easier for the blind client to accept himself. There is a caution that should be noted about contact. Contact in and of itself will not necessarily bring about change. The kind of association involved is the important thing. True acquaintance tends to lessen prejudice. The more sustained the acquaintance the less the prejudice. Those having closer contact perceive less difference than those who are farther away. Casual contact on the other hand may tend to only reinforce the prejudice, especially if persons are motivated to associate with the handicap for such unrealistic reasons as sympathy, vague fears, or pity.

Legislation is yet another way to create change, or at least create a stimulus for change. Legislation is at best only indirectly effective since real attitude change usually takes place through interpersonal relationships. Examples of legislative change in attitudes is the Civil Rights Act which says that it is against the law to discriminate on the basis of race and/or sex. Disabled people are still discriminated against, even though the Vocational Rehabilitation Act of 1973 has mandated such things as affirmative action in employment of the handicapped. Legislation such as this will go a long way toward creating an opportunity for the change of negative attitudes to more positive ones.

Psychotherapy or counseling is still another way as an individual approach but it is not easily adapted to large group situations. A particular theoretical approach to counseling that seems to be the most helpful in working with the blind individual is that approach developed by Albert Ellis called Rational Emotive Therapy (Ellis, 1962). This particular approach seems to be consistent in bringing about some change in irrational thinking, especially regarding the principles of self-inclusion and general inclusion. Ellis's theory basically teaches a person to replace irrational or "nutty" ideas with more logical and rational ones. The two principles previously discussed usually lead a person into "awfulizing" or "catastrophising," that is they are saying to themselves "ain't it awful." Ellis's approach would be to say "no, it's not awful, it's unfortunate and/or undesirable that I am blind but it is not awful because I can still work, I can still love, I can still play, etc."

There is a group of counseling or counselor attitudes which are very important for the professional rehabilitation worker of the blind if he is to bring about positive change.

Counselor Attitudes

Research on Simulating Experience

Research has shown several things regarding attitudinal formation and change. General social contact between the nondisabled and disabled which results in increased factual knowledge of the disabled leads to a more generalized tolerance and fundamental acceptance of handicapped persons (Vrie and Smith, 1970). The attitude of the counselor toward the disabled population was more important than the counselor's knowledge of counseling theory or therapeutic skills in bringing about positive therapeutic outcome for the client (Anderson, 1968). Based on these two research findings, it would appear that several positive attitudes would be desirable for the counselor to hold. Rogers, as early as 1951, discussed three of these positive professional counseling attitudes in working with all people, and they are especially pertinent to working with the disabled, most especially with the blind. Rogers called these three attitudes the therapeutic triad (Rogers, 1951). They are referred to also as core conditions or dimensions but they are basically personal and professional positive attitudes. They are empathy, respect or positive regard, and genuineness. Truax and Carkhuff (1967) and Carkhuff and Berenson (1967) have added several other positive dimensions which they feel are necessary in the counseling relationship. One of these is concreteness of expression.

Empathy — Comes from the German, *Einfühling* which means "feeling into." "This is the ability to sense a client's private world as if it were your own but without ever losing the 'as/if' quality. This is empathy and this seems essential to counseling. It is the ability to sense the client's anger, fear or confusion as if it were your own, yet without your own anger, fear or confusion getting bound into it, it is the condition we are trying to decide" (Rogers, 1961). It has also been expressed by Shertzer and Stone (1968) as the apprehension of the emotions of another without feeling completely (as in sympathy) what he feels.

Respect or Positive Regard — Has its origin in the respect which the individual has for himself. He cannot respect the feelings and experiences of others if he cannot respect his own feelings and experiences. The communication of respect appears to shadow the isolation of the individual and to establish a basis for empathy. There are strong indications that the communication of human warmth and understanding are the principal vehicles for communicating respect. There are three critical components involved in the communication of warmth. These are the helper's commitment, his effort to understand, and spontaneity (Carkhuff and Berenson, 1967).

Genuineness — The degree to which one person is functionally integrated in the context of his relationship with another, such that there is an absence of conflict or inconsistency between his total experience, his awareness, and his overt communication, with his congruence in the relationship. In short, the base for the entire therapeutic process is the establishment of a genuine relationship between helper and client. The degree to which the helper can be honest with himself and thus with the client establishes this base

(Carkhuff and Berenson, 1967).

Concreteness — Concreteness of expression is a variable which is largely under the helper's direct control and involves the fluent, direct, and complete expression of specific feelings and experiences by both helper and client regardless of their emotional content. This dimension appears to serve at least three important functions. These functions are the following:

1. The helper's concreteness ensures that his response does not become too far removed emotionally from the client's feelings and experiences.

2. Concreteness encourages the helper to be more accurrate in his understanding of the client and thus misunderstanding can be clarified and corrections made when the feelings and experiences are stated in specific terms.

3. The client is directly influenced to attend specifically to the problem areas and emotional conflicts (Carkhuff and Berenson, 1967).

Dynamic Functions of the Essential Attitudes

There are several dynamic functions of these core conditions or attitudes. These are the following, according to Carkhuff and Berenson (1967):

The facilitative stimulus complex of high amounts of these conditions or attitudes elicits client's exploration of anxiety laden material.

The anxiety reduction which takes place when the client explores himself in the context of high level of facilitative conditions or attitudes is reinforcing.

Helpers who provide high levels of these attitudes or conditions become personally potent reinforcers for the client. The high levels elicit a high degree of reciprocally positive affects of the client.

In general these attitudes or conditions help to shadow the client's experience of isolation and hopelessness.

Counseling Techniques

Techniques That Become Unimportant

Literature regarding theoretical approaches to counseling, psychotherapy, and communication lists several techniques to help communicate these attitudes or basic conditions of helping. Many of these techniques do not help or can be confusing in working with the blind individual. Some of these are as follows:

Body Language — As a helper, since the blind person cannot see the helping person — then the body language of the counselor is of no consequence. Also, body language of the client should not be taken too seriously. Many blind people have some unusual, if not unnatural, body movements. These mannerisms are not necessarily indicative of emotional or feeling states or nonverbal communication.

Eye Contact — Is another technique that is stressed as being important in counseling relationships with most people. However, the blind cannot perceive whether or not there is eye contact with the person speaking to them. Eye contact, in and of itself, is therefore useless. However, eye contact from another perspective is still important because when speaking to a blind person it is best to always face him directly. If their hearing is intact they can be very perceptive about whether or not you are facing them just by the tone and volume of the voice. They may feel, if you are not facing them directly, that you have become distracted or that you are bored in communicating with them.

The Physical Arrangements — Of the counseling office are also stressed as important for most people, especially regarding such things as furniture, lighting, and decor. Physical arrangements in working with the totally blind individual are of no consequence because the person cannot see these physical arrangements and cannot be therefore made to feel more comfortable or less distracted because of the physical arrangements of the office. It is important in terms of client comfort, however, to observe several principles of good physical arrangements such as having a comfortable chair for the client and putting the client in a position where he is not in direct heat or air conditioning. Also it is a good idea to keep in mind the fact that many blind people do have some light perception and it may be uncomfortable for them to face directly into sunlight or bright electric light.

Facial Expression — Is another area which is stressed as important for the counselor in communicating with the client. The blind client will not be able to see the facial expressions of the counselor. The counselor should be very careful in making interpretations of some affective or emotional state from the client's facial expression since many blind people have facial expressions which are not necessarily indicative of some state of anxiety or apprehension or other emotional content.

Silence — Is an occurrence that takes place in many counseling relationships and many authors feel that silence can be a constructive thing if handled well by the professional. Silence can be very confusing for any client, and even more so for the blind since visual cues are meaningless in communicating with him.

These are some techniques that probably do not have as great an impact in working with the blind client as they do with the sighted individual; however, while these become somewhat unimportant there are others that become even more important.

Techniques That Become Even More Important

Tone of Voice — The inflection, the clarity, and the vocabulary that is used in communicating with the blind person is extremely important.

Physical Contact — Is also extremely important since that is one way that the blind individual can sense caring and affection for him. These are best communicated through a good firm handshake, touching the person — like a pat on the back or placing a hand on the client's hand — or other socially acceptable types of physical contact.

Verbal Expression — Becomes extremely important for the blind person and the professional worker should explain in detail if necessary to make sure that the blind individual is getting the full benefit of the communicatioı..

Correct Information — Is extremely important in working with the blind and the correct verbalization of this information is therefore extremely important. Professional workers with the blind would be wise not to try to avoid words like see, look, show, view, movies, pictures, scenes, read, etc. Many blind people use these words themselves, but more important for the professional is the fact that the professional should be genuine and use the words that the counselor would use in his normal communication. The avoidance of such words could be interpreted by the blind person as a sympathetic sensitivity to his disability and would make him feel somewhat less than accepted in the counseling relationship.

Other Counseling Considerations

Professional workers with the blind should be willing, ready, and able to explore any and all areas with the blind client, no matter how naive it may appear. Professional workers should be very careful not to be influenced by some of the negative attitudes that have been discussed previously in this chapter. There are many cases on record where blind people have achieved things that society had said could not be done by a blind person.

One area in which naivete may loom as a formidable obstacle in communicating with the blind individual is that of sexuality. This is especially true of the congenitally blind. All one has to do is to imagine all the information that the blind person does not get from sources that are readily available to the sighted individual as he is going through his formative years. Some of these sources would be such things as adult magazines, adult books, X-rated movies, and nature. These sources are of little or no use to the blind individual simply because he has never seen them. The assumption that a professional worker might make can oftentimes be erroneous, especially in discussing topics that are dealing with sexuality. In the February 1976 issue of *Playboy* there was an article about a local radio station in the Philadelphia area that is broadcasting popular sex books and magazines that are not available in braille or on record. These programs were well received by the 1,300 blind persons who were the only audience because they had special radio receivers to catch the broadcast. This particular type of programming has been arranged by the Radio Information Center for the Blind in Philadelphia, Pennsylvania. The RICB said that the response has been generally favorable and requests received extend from such books as *Fear of Flying* and *The Joy of Sex* to hard-core pornography. Counselors would do well to not impose their own value system on the blinded individual who does not have ready access to such information.

Conclusion

It is important to recognize as professional workers in rehabilitation of the blind that attitudes can influence our behavior. It would be desirable for professional workers to be aware of their motives and attitudes because, whether they like it or not, they are a model for shaping the attitudes of all those with whom they come in contact. People, both nondisabled and disabled alike, will perceive their attitudes about their work and the people with whom they work. If the professional worker is prejudiced he will foster prejudice. If the professional worker is accepting, empathic, and genuine, then he will foster acceptance and the positive adjustment of his clients to blindness and to their whole being.

Selected References

Anderson, J. F.: *The Relationship Between Leadership Training in Group Dynamics and the Development of Groups among Disadvantaged Youth.* Unpublished manuscript, Eugene, University of Oregon, 1968.

Carkhuff, R. R. and Berenson, B. L.: *Beyond Counseling and Therapy.* New York, HR & W, 1967.

Cull, J. G.: Psychological adjustment to blindness. In Cull, J. G. and Hardy, R. E. (Eds.): *Social and Rehabilitation Services for the Blind.*

Springfield, Thomas, 1972.

Ellis, A.: *Reason and Emotion in Psychotherapy.* New York, Lyle Stuart, 1962.

Hemingway, E. G.: *Death In the Afternoon.* New York, Scribner, 1932.

Obermann, L. E.: *History of Vocational Rehabilitation in America.* Minneapolis, Minnesota, Denison, 1965.

Playboy Magazine, February 1976.

Rogers, C. R.: *On Becoming a Person.* Boston, HM, 1961.

Rogers, C. R.: *Client Centered Therapy.* Cambridge, Massachusetts, Riverside Press, 1951.

Sartain, A. Q. et al.: *Psychology: Understanding Human Behavior.* New York, McGraw, 1962.

Sherif, Muzafer et. al.: *Attitudes and Attitude Change: The Social Judgement — Involvement Approach.*

Shertzer, B. and Stone, S. C.: *Fundamentals of Counseling.* Boston, HM, 1968.

Truax, C. B. and Carkhuff, R. R.: *Toward Effective Counseling and Psychotherapy: Training and Practice.* Chicago, Aldine, 1967.

Vrie, R. E. and Smith, A. H.: The effects of peer contact on attitudes toward disabled college students. *Journal of Applied Rehabilitation Counseling, 1*(4):3-9, 1970.

Wallace, J. H.: Attitudes and blindness. In Hardy, R. E. and Cull, J. G. (Eds.): *Social and Rehabilitation Services For the Blind.* Springfield, Thomas, 1972.

CHAPTER 17

IMPLICATIONS FOR REHABILITATION OF BLIND INDIVIDUALS

WILLIAM T. COPPAGE

GENERALIZATIONS concerning the current relationships which exist between ophthalmologists and rehabilitation programs for blind people are difficult and perhaps risky to make. These relationships do vary widely among the communities throughout the United States. In many areas there is convincing evidence of very close cooperation and in others there is still much to be done in cultivating a desirable climate in which roles are clearly defined, understood, and adhered to.

It would seem advisable at this point to take a look at some specific areas of misunderstanding which have surfaced during the years and some approaches which have been employed to successfully resolve problems.

Ophthalmologists have been known to become overzealous in dealing with their patients and have prescribed for blind people beyond their medical needs. They have prescribed for educational, social, physical (other than eye health), and other kinds of needs. Although well intentioned, the doctor does not always realize that he cannot be all things to all people anymore than can the state rehabilitation agency. An illustration of this point would be the recommending of large print books where the youngster can get along perfectly well with regular print books as long as the light is appropriate and the material is held close enough to be seen. By doing this, the child has access to a much wider variety of reading materials at far less cost than in the case of where large print is used. There are known instances of doctors advising parents to send their visually handicapped child to the state residential school for the blind. This seldom is necessary or advisable if blindness or a severe visual loss is the only handicap. Most local school systems now have programs adequate to cope with the special education needs of these children. Where recommendations like these are made, the impact on the client and family is most significant since the ophthalmologist is the one on whom trust has been placed and the service agency staff are not able to work effectively in the face of recommendations from physicians. Working together, however, the ophthalmologists and the state rehabilitation agency can bring to bear the various resources needed to effectively cope with a patient/client's individual problems.

Some ophthalmologists have offered false hope to blind people with regard to treatment or sight restoration. Most blind people will refuse rehabilitative services if they believe the loss of sight is temporary. A successful rehabilitation program can seldom be provided to an individual who believes that his sight will be restored.

In some communities ophthalmologists do not understand low vision aids programs and become resentful when a patient is referred to another ophthalmologist who specializes in the prescription of special optical aids. Although many ophthalmologists are trained in this specialty, some are not and efforts are being made to help them understand that agencies for the blind are not pirating their patients for other ophthalmologists. In Virginia, for example, working agreements are developed with ophthalmologists who are trained to provide the specialized examinations and who are in a position to devote the extra time which is a necessary part of such examinations in the effort to make this service available to all who need them. Some doctors provide these examinations through low vision aids clinics and others directly from the office.

Many states have reporting laws which require that ophthalmologists and others who determine an individual to be within the legal definition of blindness report the patient's name and other specified data to the state agency for the blind. Most state registers are incomplete primarily due to the fact that blind persons are not reported. Occasionally, an ophthalmologist fails to report a patient's name unless he feels the individual cannot assume financial responsibility for his service. Data contained on the state registers is kept confidential and agencies do not insist on providing any services when patients indicate than none are desired. Also, some ophthalmologists do report individuals as legally blind but either fail to supply information on the amount of vision or use a phrase — "unable to determine." This creates a problem at times in making individuals eligible for programs such as the American Printing House Quota. I would suggest that ophthalmologists could assist significantly by putting in a specific measurement of vision even if it is based on a calculated judgment or an estimate.

A few additional problems which have been identified include the following: (1) Ophthalmologists as well as optometrists need to be aware of the fact that their professional differences at times create real problems for blind persons and for agencies attempting to serve the public. This is exemplified in the Rehabilitation Regulations which provide that "the State plan shall provide that in all cases of visual impairment a visual examination will be provided by a physician skilled in the diseases of the eye or by an optometrist, whichever the individual may select." (2) There is a growing trend to encourage individuals with limited vision to drive automobiles using special optical aids, particularly telescopic devices with very restricted visual fields. Initially this effort seemed to be centered among optometrists but more recently some opthalmologists have become involved. This has been creating considerable difficulty for rehabilitation personnel and other professionals since some persons are encouraged to drive when it may not be completely safe for them to do so. Again, solutions are not easy but I believe that advice from the ophthalmologist would be of considerable assistance to service agencies. (3) Ophthalmologists sometimes complain of low fees for operations and treatment procedures. The fees, however, are often beyond the direct control of agencies requiring the service since fees are established by other state or federal agencies.

Let us spend a little time now looking at the current state of the art as it exists in some parts of the country and perhaps should exist in the rest of the nation. State agency boards, commissions, and advisory groups contain ophthalmologists among their membership. Where this is so, ophthalmologists are afforded an opportunity to observe and understand agency programs and services. Many times this knowledge is communicated to their fellow colleagues at professional meetings, civic clubs, and social gatherings. Also state agencies participate in programs of local, state, and national ophthalmological societies, and in many places the agency also displays an exhibit at conventions or special meetings held by ophthalmologists. Some states attempt to communicate in other ways such as periodic mailings of special materials including public information folders for distribution to visually impaired patients, reporting forms, copies of state reporting laws, etc. Another effective approach which is being used in some communities is the inclusion of classroom lectures from the state rehabilitation agency in departments of ophthalmology at medical schools. Residents from these schools often include tours of rehabilitation facilities as part of the curriculum. Increasingly, agencies for the blind are contracting with ophthalmologists to assist with staff development programs including orientation and lectures for new agency employees.

Personal visits to ophthalmologists have long been the practice of rehabilitation counselors and other field workers for the purpose of better acquainting the physicians with services provided for visually handicapped people by local service agencies for the blind. This may be done during a visit to the doctor's office or during a meeting at some community civic organization.

Obviously, only the surface has been scratched in looking at a few things which are taking place today; however, it is encouraging to observe that, through better communications, better working relationships do now exist. By working together we can and will reinforce one another in our respective roles to help visually impaired individuals cope with their special problems.

References

1. Hardy, R. E. and Cull, J. G.: *Social and Rehabilitation Services for the Blind*. Springfield, Thomas, 1972.
2. Vail, Derrick: *The Truth About Your Eyes*. New York, FS & G, 1950.

CHAPTER 18

THE HUMAN GUIDE

C. WARREN BLEDSOE

GUIDING blind people is not a science. There is, however, a technique which rises to the point of being an art when learned with sensitivity to the needs of others. It is almost invariably learned behavior. It comes naturally to very few sighted people who encounter blind ones. Without that learned behavior there is bound to be tension between a blind person and a sighted companion when doing things together — little skirmishes, awkwardness, frustrations, embarrassments.

We know that the wise have analyzed this problem for centuries when we read in the "Analects" how Confucius handled it.[1] He is pictured carefully guiding his sightless music teacher down a flight of steps, seating him on his mat, and telling him who were present in the room. To a visitor who inquired, "Is it the rule to tell these things to the music master?" Confucius solemnly replied, "This is certainly the rule for those who guide the blind." By this we may assume that along with his other great qualities, Confucius was one of those people who by inherent sensitivity was a great sighted companion of blind people, as we sometimes find them depicted in the literature about blindness.

In the early twentieth century a notable American worker for the blind received similar tributes. This was Mr. Charles Campbell, who had learned to guide blind people from his incomparable, blind father, Sir Francis Campbell.[2] Charles Campbell initiated many constructive activities for blind people in this

---

[1]Ross, Ishbel: *Journey Into Light.* New York, 1951, p. 22.
[2]Francis Joseph Campbell (1832-1914) was a world-famous blind educator of the blind. Born an American, in middle life he was founder of the Royal Normal College and Academy of Music for the Blind in Great Britain. He was knighted by King Edward VII.

country. Helen Keller said, "Wonderful as Mr. Campbell's work was, I shall always think of him as he was in the intimacies of life. When he stepped on the platform beside me all the nervousness and apprehension vanished."[3]

It is impossible to measure how much public support came to blind people as a result of Helen Keller's lack of nervousness and apprehension on the stage. In Japan alone during the 1930s one of her public speaking campaigns netted 34 million yen (17 million dollars) for the blind people of Japan.

A French Academy authority on Montaigne, Pierre Villey, who was blind, is responsible for a much quoted panegyric describing people whom he termed the "élite" where blindness is concerned. Villey wrote the following:

> They know without being told that to oblige a blind man, they must not always act for him, but without any affectation, help him to take as large a share as he can himself in the common action, so that he may have the satisfaction of doing things with others and like others and even, in his turn, for others. Their attention, although vigilant, does not weigh on him, so natural is it and so discreet. They guess instinctively what is difficult for the blind man and they do it for him without talking about it, and almost without thinking about it. They understand that when guiding him, they do not need to warn him about the various things on the way, but to make him guess them by their movements. They give him all the help that is necessary, but only the help necessary. They talk to him about everything, even about blindness, without the slightest embarrassment. They have that marvelous art of divination, which is called tact, a mysterious mixture made of the keenest intelligence and the most delicate kindness.[4]

Most of us are not like that. Our ordinary, close, personal, social amenities are based on the assumption that our companions can see. Richard Hoover, M.D. once said one of the things that makes it possible for us to get along with each other is the large number of ways in which we are similar, ways in which we assume that others are like us. A prime example of this is the assumption that the other fellow has eyesight. Assumptions

---

[3]*Outlook for the Blind*, 30:8, 1936.
[4]Villey, Pierre: *The World of the Blind*. London, 1930.

like this, however, trip us up when we encounter those who are markedly different in this respect. Even those of us who are old hands with blindness are forever forgetting that in one respect blind people are not like us. Their very capabilities make us forget that they are different in not being able to see.

This is keenly, even smartingly, observed by blind people, as it was in an incident related to me at Dibble Army General Hospital during World War II. A blinded soldier, a country boy, had been guided by a sighted corpsman through the ramifications of the enormous hospital to the psychiatrist's office. The purpose of the expedition was to check on the blinded soldier's wits. In this connection the psychiatrist posed the question, "Can this fellow who guided you down here see?" The blinded soldier said, "I speck he can." The psychiatrist said, "Why do you think so?" The blinded soldier said, "Because I ran into three things coming down here and he didn't run into any."

The sighted guide of the blind individual with or without experience frequently forgets how wide his blind companion's shoulders are.

I am the butt of another ancedote, further illustrating such forgetfulness. Mr. Louis Rives was the victim.

Mr. Rives, who is totally without sight, is not only a brilliant lawyer but an expert mechanic. For several years he and I had been driving to work together. About two weeks ago on leaving our offices we discovered I had a flat tire. Mr. Rives wanted to get home quickly and knew that my mechanical skill was nil, so he took over the changing of the tire. The jack was one of those clever devices, in three parts when stored, which combines its utilitarian purpose with the diabolical aspects of a Chinese puzzle. Between flats I always forget how it is supposed to go together and it takes me a small chunk of eternity to assemble it. It is particularly deceptive to the eye. After exploring it by touch, Mr. Rives assembled it in a jiffy, put it to use, and unscrewed the lugs on the wheel containing the flat. Meanwhile I, burning to be useful, had taken the spare out of the trunk and placed it just behind him so that when he stood back he fell over it. (Fortunately without bodily damage.)

He was very forgiving, merely saying, "It's your sighted friends you have to look out for."

I have known Mr. Rives forgiveness for nearly two decades, having gone to work for him at HEW in 1957. The first time I had lunch with him, we went to the office cafeteria. As we went foraging through the line, a plate of blueberry pie suddenly acquired life of its own, jumped from my grasp, and took for its mark Mr. Rives's pearl-gray suit. He appeared entirely unruffled and now claims he cannot remember the episode.

Such poise and kindness should bring out the best in us and make us feel we should give the best we have in guiding and all it implies in personal relationships with blind people. However, it is easy to grow careless, especially when associating with extremely agile blind people who lull you into forgetting they cannot see. This is why some of us have tried to ease the way for both blind people and their sighted companions by setting down some rules for guiding. They have been refined several times, but always with a view to keeping them as clear and practical as possible.

A few explanations should accompany these rules. They are quite simple, at least to read, but they are not childishly simple to apply. They take thought and practice. They came into existence because of the difficulty not of understanding but of *actually remembering* to do what we ought to do in the way of courtesy toward blind people. This is quite different from going through the motions of finding out what those things are without acting them out.

The whirlwind of experience with blind and sighted people at Valley Forge General Hospital during World War II was reaped and turned to purpose by Dr. Hoover and Mr. Russell Williams. Early in the effort there was much talk about an unstructured program. A theory was advanced that blinded soldiers would learn best the ways of blindness without teaching, especially from sighted instructors, and that there was a good deal to be said for learning by bumping into things. Among our sighted medical corpsmen, one was a clever cartoonist. Another was a pudgy loquacious fellow, a little slow to action. One morning there appeared on the bulletin board of one of the eye wards a cartoon depicting a blinded soldier seeing stars as his head sharply struck a door which was ajar. Looking on was the heavy boy, hands in pockets and feet crossed, saying, "Oh, that reminds me, on entering a ward, you will find two doors that extend out from the wall a little."

Dr. Hoover decided to capitalize on this spontaneous artistic talent, and a handbook emerged with illustrations by the artist corpsman. It went far toward making the people at Valley Forge Hospital reasonably thoughtful with regard to blind people. Today's rules on guiding have descended from that handbook, having been done over and published several times once by the Veterans Administration and more recently by the American Association of Workers for the Blind. The last revision was for inclusion in a handbook for volunteers. It appears as an appendix to this paper.

It will be the people who work around ophthalmologists (receptionists, doormen, secretaries, office nurses) who will find the instructions most helpful. Because of medical and surgical obligations upon ophthalmologists few of them will spend much time acting as guides. We workers for the blind understand that. Nevertheless, it may be said that a more intimate familiarity with blind individuals might cause ophthalmologists to sleep better. They would find, as most of us do with things we dread, that when close to them, the dread lessens. To know blind people as a guide can be very rewarding.

Every human being has in his make-up not only common items of constitution, even in specific diseases, but also unique strengths and elements of construction. In this singularity lies the special magic of each man, woman, and child. Human charm, which we never quite understand, is almost as important in binding society together as are the sensations we all have in common. By the magnetism of individual personalities opposites are drawn together. One of the great disservices which the pseudo-Freudians (not the leader himself) have done to society is to suggest that all personal attractions are somehow akin to the erotic. It might be more accurate to say they are akin to what religious folk call the *holy spirit*.

Copybook wisdom of work for the blind has long held that

each blind person is an individual. Blind people are not a class. Seldom if ever have I gotten to know a blind person who did not have the individual magnetism of which I speak, whether the person was very complex or very simple.

Among the very simple was an old man in a domiciliary for aged blind veterans who said, "Tell General Bradley I need a chair without arms, because when I play my mouth organ the music goes through me from my fingers to my toes." To this he added, "You take the simplest man on earth. Sometimes he knows something no one else knows."

In contrast, a brilliant blind veteran noted for a sharp stiletto in repartee, said to his nurse, "'Skeezix,' is that all you can think of to call me? Here I've been crawling over the battlefield, over dead bodies for you people. You might at least call me young man." He needed extended plastic surgery and had a long stay in the hospital. Once he was introduced by the chief of ophthalmology of the hospital to a visiting general and the eye chief said proudly, "This young fellow has been with us eighteen months." To this the young patient said, "And don't think it ain't been charmin'!" I am sorry to say that this seemed to hurt the eye chief's feelings.

In their commitment to the saving of sight ophthalmologists sometimes seem to take such surgical humor a little harder than they should. Perhaps those of us in work for the blind accept such word play too readily. A sense of humor oftentimes seems the most important ingredient in adjustment to blindness. For physicians, Sir William Osler himself set the example of "laughing that I may not weep."

Another important ingredient for the human guide is illustrated in the colloquy between the eye chief and the blinded soldier just mentioned. In rehabilitation, even what we usually think is pardonable pride must be restrained. There are some professionals whose vanity the public is very ready to excuse. We pardon baseball players, actors, soldiers, cooks, and courtesans for showing plainly they think they have done a good job. Undertakers and wardens of penitentiaries learn early that if they show themselves puffed up over a performance, they are sure to be deflated. There is an appreciation spectrum along which physicians, dentists, and people in the so-called helping professions are ranged. In this spectrum, no doubt, ophthalmologists are a little closer to the end occupied by Zsa Zsa Gabor, whereas workers for the blind are a little closer to the end occupied by the commissioner of Internal Revenue. Yet the glamor that comes from being associated with the saving of life and relief of suffering, though diminished, does not evaporate entirely even when blindness occurs, at least in the minds of the patient's family and the public. The prestige of physicians can be an enormous help in improving attitudes toward blind people. At least two golden ages in work for the blind have evolved through the interest and intervention of ophthalmologists. One occurred under the leadership of Dr. Thomas Rhodes Armitage in Britain between 1872 and 1914. The other was brought to pass by the Army ophthalmologists in the United States during World War II.

In summary, there are several aspects of the ophthalmologist's role in work for the blind. The most important element with which he may begin is by making sure that everyone around him is knowledgeable in regard to special courtesies which make blindness easier. Proper guiding is fundamental. If he can make sure that the patient's family understands this, it can be the opening wedge for acceptance of services for the blind. This is an important hurdle, not only for the patient but for the physician. The patient has a better chance of making the hurdle if his ophthalmologist has learned to take it skillfully in behalf of the patient, however much he may deplore and feel chagrin over the loss of sight.

APPENDIX

Suggestions for Guiding Blind Individuals

The guiding of blind individuals is a personal service which sighted people are called upon to give. It has been noticed that most people find a certain awkwardness in the role of guide, which arises from their lack of knowledge of effective techniques of handling the situation. To assist in relieving this uncertainty, some governing principles have been set down from time to time as follows:

1. Always try to remember that a blind person cannot see. This fact is apt to escape the associates of blind people as they gain a familiarity with the effectiveness which is possible for the blind, and lose the impression that blindness means helplessness. There is no magic to the effectiveness of blind people, and it depends heavily upon securing from seeing people information which cannot possibly be gained without the aid of human eye, or which could be gained by touch, but only with embarrassment, as, for example, information that there are both biscuits and rolls on a bread tray. Openness, directness, and unobtrusiveness should govern the imparting of such information.

2. Ask the blind person to take your arm. Never take his arm and propel him by the elbow. Show him where your elbow is by touching his arm with it.

3. Ordinarily walk half a pace ahead of the blind person. In going up and down steps, or into dangerous places, keep one pace ahead of him. After some practice with you he will be able to know he has reached steps by the movement of your arm.

4. Always tell the blind person whom you have not guided before when you come to steps.

5. When going into narrow or dangerous places, always go ahead. The blind person is at his poorest when you try to get him to precede you. Never seize him by the upper arm from behind and shove him around.

6. Coming to a small irregularity in the terrain over which he might stumble, tell him about it.

7. Be careful at all times not to let his opposite side bump into door frames and obstructions. This will require extreme watchfulness.

8. If it is necessary for the blind person to make some slight movement to the left or right, to get out of the way or maneuver into positions, direct him orally. Once again, don't shove him.

9. A diagonal approach to a curb, or flight of steps, is awkward for a blind person who is following a guide. Take the trouble to square off and approach at right angles.

10. The good guide is inconspicuous. He doesn't take over and run things on a trip to the bank or drugstore. When someone speaks to a blind person

through his guide, the guide may direct the conversation of the clerk to the blind individual. This will usually be sufficient.

11. At all times picture carefully what move the blind person is about to make, in order that exact directions may be given. Be helpful by looking ahead and anticipating. Especially avoid mixing right and left, particularly when you face the blind person and his right becomes your left.

12. Give an honest play-by-play account of what you are seeing, as desired or required.

13. When you guide a blind person into a place of public assembly, be sure he understands his location, especially if you leave him for a few moments. It is better under such circumstances to establish a point of contact, such as a counter, table, chair or wall.

14. In a place of public assembly, where there is confusion, a blind person needs more help than in familiar surroundings. Many of the little things he does for himself with ease in his own environment will be difficult in a different environment. Give him the help he needs in a case like this.

15. The expressions "over here," "down there," and "right here" should be used sparingly. Use instead "let me show you" to fill up the time lag until you establish actual physical contact between the blind individual and the object you are trying to help him find. One way to establish this contact is by oral direction, carefully and precisely worded. Another is by tapping the object sought, in which case, as you tap it, you may say "it's there." A third means is by saying, "let me take your hand," and placing it on the object he wishes to use.

16. At times the most practical method of maneuvering a blind person into position is to drop his arm, move to the spot where you want him to go, and say "come toward me," letting your voice guide him. This will not work, of course, when the blind person has a hearing defect which involves an inability to detect the direction from which sound proceeds. Persons having frequent contact with the blind should be alerted to this type of hearing impairment.

17. When giving directions, or in any other conversation with the blind individual, speak no more loudly than necessary, speak distinctly, and direct your words to the blind person alone.

18. In a narrow passage, such as those leading to dining and Pullman cars on trains, it is sometimes not practical for the blind person walking behind you to hold your arm. He may then put his hands on your shoulder, or in the middle of your back, touching it lightly.

19. In guiding a blind person to a chair, one method is to bring him to a point at which he touches it and knows which direction it faces. It will then be a simple matter for him to examine it with his hands, pull it out from a table for himself if this is necessary, and handle his own actions in whatever way he prefers.

20. In entering an automobile, a blind person can engineer his own actions if he is told in which direction the vehicle is facing. One hand is placed on

the door handle and the other on the top of the car. The situation is then familiar enough to suggest the whole picture to him. If he becomes confused, further information can be given. Not more than one person should take over in a case like this.

21. If any or all of the above items annoy the blind person, disregard them and guide him the way he likes to be guided, unless you have time and authority to investigate his objections and explain to him the reasons for your way. If, after such an explanation, he still prefers variations of method, accede to his wishes.

22. Be prepared for the blind person to make direct statements concerning any awkward situations which develop. Usually, these will be in a humorous vein, which will indicate that he wants to put you at your ease. It is safe to follow his lead in an attitude of this kind, and let him keep the lead. A contrasting sharpness of utterance and reaction to an awkward situation may indicate he feels you are an individual whom he can trust sufficiently to relieve himself of frustration by expressing annoyance at his difficulties in your presence.

23. If you find that you cannot cope with your own feeling toward blindness, and are regularly called upon to guide blind people, try to get in touch with some well-seasoned blind person, who is engaged in rehabilitation work; then talk with him or her about your feelings. Such people are glad to share with you the attitudes which have made it possible for them to face the hard realities of the situation. They will be glad to assist you in being a friend to blind people without morbid emotion.*

*Adapted from material prepared by C. Warren Bledsoe, Division of Services for the Blind, Vocational Rehabilitation Administration, Department of Health, Education, and Welfare. Reprinted by American Association of Workers for the Blind, September 1966.

CHAPTER 19

ADVICE TO THE PERMANENTLY BLIND INDIVIDUAL ABOUT HIS WORK OPPORTUNITIES

William F. Gallagher

I HAVE been asked to give my advice to those permanently blinded persons about their job opportunities.

In graduate school and social work, it was drilled into us that we should never give advice — it is a poor professional practice and does not really help the client. So, as most professional persons do, I am breaking away from what I was taught and I shall discuss with you some of the advice I would give to a blind person who is being counseled regarding his vocational future.

My first bit of advice to a blind person is that he should be trained in all of the necessary skills and techniques to function independently. He should work hard to gain insight about his feelings toward blindness and whether it interferes with his relationships with people. He should know what he can and cannot do, and when he cannot do something, he should be willing to accept assistance. However, whenever he can he should do for himself and not allow other persons to do for him or he will keep slipping deeper and deeper into a dependent pattern that will develop until he is totally dependent upon others for everything.

A totally blind person should understand the advantages and disadvantages of the cane and dog guide and should decide to use whichever he is most comfortable with. If he is going to use a cane, he should be trained by a mobility specialist who has been trained in one of the graduate programs in our universities; there are approximately eight or nine universities offering such training in orientation and mobility teaching at the graduate level. If he should decide to use a dog guide, then he should make application to one of the more reliable dog guide schools. All of the universities that have courses in mobility teaching and all of the dog guide schools are listed in the *Directory of Agencies Serving the Visually Handicapped in the U.S.*, which is published by the American Foundation for the Blind.

The blind person should be familiar with all of the reading and writing communication tools; he should know what is available, how to use them, and most importantly be comfortable using them in front of sighted persons. So many times the blind person uses braille, the abacus, the Optacon® and other reading devices at home but feels uneasy in using them in a public place.

A blind person should work hard to develop his techniques in daily living skills. There are too many daily living skills to list at this time, but they include eating, grooming, leisure time activities, etc.

I strongly recommend that the blind person practice his oral communication, such as looking at a person when talking to him, maintaining a good relaxed posture and facial and body expression — all of these will assist the sighted person to feel at ease with him. Many employers often say, "I was very uncomfortable when interviewing a blind person. He did not look at me; he looked straight ahead or up in the air, or in another direction. If I am uncomfortable with him, then so will be my other employees."

Many capable, qualified blind persons have lost job opportunities solely because of poor oral communication. This is a service that we, in the field of business, have neglected. It is important to know when to speak and when not to speak in a conversation and if the other party is looking at you or is looking or talking to someone else in the room.

If a blind person is relaxed and comfortable in routine conversations with sighted persons, then he should also feel comfortable in competing in vocational settings.

I would advise the permanently blinded person to know his trade; in fact, it would not hurt if he knew it better than his sighted fellow worker.

The blind person should not be limited to looking for jobs

just within his own neighborhood or city. If work opportunities are better in another city or state, he should have the confidence to move. As we all know, we are a moving generation and, by having a work experience in another city or state, the blind person will have the chance to grow in his job.

I would advise the blind person to be active in his leisure time — try to compete in a recreational setting with sighted persons from the neighborhood. Become active and involved in community affairs. This will help not only the community but it will also help to build good emotional health.

As you well know, the majority of blind persons lose their sight as adults, therefore, these persons need comprehensive rehabilitation programs. Trying to give newly blinded persons rehabilitation in a piecemeal fashion does not work — it only frustrates and confuses them.

Before rehabilitation can begin, the newly blinded person must accept the fact that he is blind and that he is going to remain blind. Too often we see false hope by the newly blinded person — he is always hoping that he will regain his eyesight, either through modern medical techniques or a miracle. Only after he has accepted the permanency of his blindness will he settle in for total rehabilitation.

There are approximately fifty state and private rehabilitation centers for the blind listed in the American Foundation for the Blind's directory.

I feel that the person who is working and then becomes blind should have the opportunity to be rehabilitated before making his decision about leaving work and accepting a disability retirement. Too many times the newly blinded person makes his decision before he knows what he can do as a blind person. Also, the company may not be sure about what he can do and, meaning well, place him on medical retirement. Most companies have excellent pension plans but an employee who becomes blind should not use such a plan until he has to do so. My advice to the newly blinded person is "take time out from work — go on a leave of absence — enter a rehabilitation center, then when you have completed this program, decide whether you want to return to work or if you would prefer to accept a disability retirement."

I have heard the newly blinded person in a rehabilitation center say, "If I had only known what I could do as a blind person, I never would have given up my job." He stated that he just did not know how he would function as a blind person and that the company for whom he worked shared this same anxiety about his work ability. By the time he had begun rehabilitation it was too late for him to return to work — he had accepted a medical retirement, the company had replaced him, and now there was just no room for him.

My advice to newly permanently blinded persons is not to make quick decisions; think it over very carefully before you decide that you cannot function as well as you had before you lost your sight. In most cases, it is not eyesight but the person's experience, knowledge, and ability that counts on the job — you lose none of this when you become blind.

If we afford people the opportunity to be rehabilitated and then return to their previous employment, we shall not have the difficult task of training or retraining them for new careers.

Each company or place of employment should have written into its medical plan (contained in the personnel practices) a clause that states that *anyone who becomes disabled at work should have the opportunity to be rehabilitated before being offered an early retirement.*

My advice to administrators of state rehabilitation programs is that you have a responsibility to see that blind men and women in your state have the opportunity for a comprehensive rehabilitation program to acquire the necessary skills and techniques to function independently, and the freedom to decide their own vocational futures.

My advice to the ophthalmological consultants is to know what blind persons can do, to know your community resources and especially those of the state rehabilitation agencies for the blind and visually handicapped. If there are private agencies for the blind in your community, know their function and purpose.

Suggested Readings

American Foundation for the Blind: *Directory of Agencies Serving the Visually Handicapped in the United States,* 18th ed. New York, Am Foun Blind, 1973.

American Foundation for the Blind: *How Does a Blind Person Get Around?* New York, Am Foun Blind, 1973.

Bauman, Mary K. and Yoder, Norman M.: *Placing the Blind and Visually Handicapped in Clerical, Industrial and Service Fields.* HEW, Vocational Rehabilitation Administration, Washington, D.C., U.S. Govt Print Office, 1965.

Bauman, Mary K. and Yoder, Norman M.: *Adjustment to Blindness Reviewed.* Springfield, Thomas, 1966.

Carroll, Thomas J.: *Blindness — What It Is, What It Does and How to Live With It.* Boston, Little, 1961.

Licht, Sidney: *Rehabilitation and Medicine.* Baltimore, Maryland, Williams & Wilkins, 1968.

Welsh, R. L.: Cognitive and psychosocial aspects of mobility training. In American Association of Workers for the Blind: *Blindness.* Washington, D.C., AAWB, 1972.

CHAPTER 20

THE EMPLOYMENT OF THE VISUALLY IMPAIRED IN THE FEDERAL GOVERNMENT

HEDWIG OSWALD

THE federal government, as the nation's largest single employer, provides employment opportunities to all disabled persons, including the blind, in positions for which they can qualify. This supports the traditional concept of assuring equal opportunity to all citizens desiring federal employment and is fully compatible with the goal of efficiency and economy in government. The program, having a solid foundation in law and presidential directives, serves to focus attention on a frequently overlooked source of valuable manpower.

Implementation of this program is the responsibility of the United States Civil Service Commission (CSC), the central personnel agency for the federal government. The commission serves as the catalyst for a nationwide effort by coordinating all program phases with federal agencies. Working through its ten regional offices and its sixty-five area offices, the CSC maintains relationships with public and private agencies who are concerned with the employment of the disabled. There are at present some 3,500 Coordinators for Selective Placement of the Disabled, representing every federal organization having personnel hiring authority.

Agency coordinators are the most important persons in the system. They are the ones who bring applicants and selecting officials together. Coordinators are in the unique position of knowing agency managers and supervisors and the kinds of jobs that need to be filled. At the same time, they rely upon the professional assistance of rehabilitation counselors in state agencies serving the blind and other disabled groups, as well as upon the assistance of the medical community. Placement efforts are directed to all groups — the moderately as well as the severely disabled. This process assures the fullest utilization of this source of needed manpower.

Most physically disabled applicants, including a majority of the visually impaired, find employment through the normal competitive procedures in the same manner as the nondisabled; however, the *severely* physically disabled — persons with disabilities of such a severe nature that they are unable to demonstrate their capabilities to obtain federal employment through the regular application and examining process — may be employed under the "expected service" provisions of a special hiring authority. This means that an individual needs only to be qualified to perform tasks of a *specific* job, not a class of positions — in other words, he is not in competition with others. Under this authority an agency may determine if a disabled applicant meets the minimum qualifications for the position, appoint him on a trial basis, and, if he is successful, convert the trial appointment to a permanent one. Another approach permits the agency to accept, from a state or Veterans Administration vocational rehabilitation counselor, a certification stating that the applicant is able to handle a particular job. Appointments under this system must be approved by the Civil Service Commission.

There has been a marked increase in the number of disabled persons employed in federal agencies throughout the various regions since the program was first initiated in 1964. As the total number of all disabled employed in federal service has increased so has the number of appointments of the visually impaired:

Year	Number of Blind Appointed
1964-1965	1
1966-1967	19
1968-1969	52
1970-1971	130
1972-1973	88

The number of visually impaired hired in 1972-1973 declined as a result of freezes on hiring; however, it should be noted that in the first three months of 1974 there was a 25 percent increase in the number of disabled employed under excepted appointment authorities.

Blindness is a serious disability but it does not mean helplessness. Today in the federal service, the blind are using their talents in administrative, technical, and professional positions as well as in the semiskilled and clerical fields. Although statistical data presently are not maintained on the number and kinds of positions of blind (or other disabled) employees within the *total* federal work force, Tables 20-I and 20-II give a general overview of pay schedules and job titles of visually impaired employees hired under the special appointing authority for the years 1964 through 1973.

TABLE 20-I

PAY SCHEDULES AT TIME OF APPOINTMENT OF
VISUALLY IMPAIRED EMPLOYEES

1964-1973

General Schedule (GS)		*Number*	
GS-1		14	
GS-2		35	
GS-3	(General Schedule positions	58	
GS-4	correspond with "white	73	
GS-5	collar" positions in	22	
GS-7	private industry.)	8	
GS-9		1	
		Subtotal	211
Wage Grade (WG)			
WG-1		17	
WG-2	(Wage Grade positions	12	
WG-3	correspond with "blue	7	
WG-4	collar" positions in	8	
WG-5	private industry.)	14	
WG-9		1	
		Subtotal	59

Postal Service (PS)

PS-1	1
PS-2	7
PS-3	8
PS-4	4
Subtotal	20

TOTAL	290

TABLE 20-II

JOB TITLES AT TIME OF APPOINTMENT OF VISUALLY IMPAIRED EMPLOYEES

1964-1973

Title	*Number*
Auto Mechanic Helper	1
Auto Worker	1
Card Punch Operator	1
Carpenter Helper	1
Clerk	25
Clerk, Accounts Maintenance	2
Clerk, Carrier	1
Clerk, Claims	22
Clerk, Dictating Machine Operator/Transcriber	16
Clerk, Mail or File	3
Clerk, Payroll	1
Clerk, Personnel Staffing	5
Clerk, Steno	1
Clerk, Supply	3
Clerk, Translator	2
Clerk-Typist	10
Commissary Stock Handler	1
Computer Aid (Trainee)	5
Computer Operator	1
Computer Programmer	8
Computer Technician	3
Custodian	3
Dark Room Aid	1
Domestic Appliance Repairer	1
Educational Therapist	1

Electrical Equipment Repairer Helper	1
Elevator Operator	1
Film Processing Handler	1
Food and Drug Technician	1
Food Service Worker	4
Gauge Checker Helper	1
Guidance Counselor	1
Health Technician	2
Helper General	1
Housekeeping Aid	2
Industrial Shop Worker	2
Information Receptionist	2
Laboratory Helper	2
Laborer	11
Laundry Worker	3
Mail Handler	15
Mathematician	1
Medical Radio Technician	3
Medical Receptionist and Transcriber	1
Meteorologist	1
Ordinance Equipment Mechanic	1
Packer	6
Personnel Management Specialist	2
Produce Attendant	2
Radiological Film Processor	1
Research Assistant	1
Social Worker	2
Special Employment Assistant	1
Taxpayer Service Representative and Tax Examiner	73
Telephone Inquiry Specialist	8
Telephone Operator	2
Trades Helper	1
X-Ray Film Processor	16
TOTAL	290

Certain agencies have discovered that some jobs often can best be performed by people with partial or total blindness and have given great impetus to the total Selective Placement Program through their efforts. The Internal Revenue Service (IRS) of the Treasury Department began in 1966 to train and employ the blind as taypayer service representatives. This training project was funded by a grant from the Rehabilitation Service Administration of the Department of Health, Education, and Welfare and has proven to be very successful. Arkansas Enterprises for the Blind, Little Rock, Arkansas, coordinates all of the training for IRS. Initially, the Internal Revenue Service was committed to employ up to one hundred blind taxpayer service representatives whose work consists primarily of answering, over the telephone, technical questions from the public concerning income taxes. As of January 1974, ninety three placements had been made with three more candidates in training. It is now anticipated this program will continue beyond the earlier established commitment of one hundred positions.

The Social Security Administration (SSA) of the Department of Health, Education, and Welfare used similar techniques in preparing blind persons for careers as telephone service representatives. The idea, which originated with a blind, double-amputee vocational rehabilitation counselor for the state of Florida, ultimately led to the implementation of a specialized training program begun in June 1969. Applicants are referred by state vocational rehabilitation offices. Those selected enter a thirteen-week training class conducted by SSA and, upon successful completion of all requirements, are appointed to telephone service representative positions.

In January 1973, the CSC launched a special project designed to employ blind men and women as information specialists in federal job information centers all across the country. Each specialist must be familiar with all facets of federal employment — how to apply for positions; qualifications standards; local and national job markets; and regulations dealing with promotions, health benefits, reduction-in-force procedures, and all the many other personnel subject areas. Blind applicants for these positions must attend a thirty-day prevocational evaluation session, which tends to predict successful graduates of the program, before proceeding on to a three-month training program conducted at the Arkansas Enterprises for the Blind. Three classes already have been graduated and their students placed into effective job roles.

The qualification standards for getting into these training programs are tough, but this is necessary. Graduates of the programs must fulfill highly disciplined roles as businessmen and women. They are expected to have what it takes to succeed — for themselves and for the sake of programs that will benefit others as well. It is significant to note again that these positions are filled not only through special appointing authorities but also through the regular competitive process.

Past years' experiences in these efforts have proven that well-qualified blind individuals, once employed, can and do perform just as well as their sighted peers — in jobs where eyesight is not an absolute requirement. Forward looking changes during current years about the kinds of work that can be performed by the visually impaired have helped. Job restructuring and the development of hardware aids have greatly broadened employment prospects.

This type of philosophy can be further broadened to include *all* types of disabilities be they physical or mental, for, once employed, a majority of disabled individuals satisfactorily perform the duties of their positions. Whatever problems do arise appear to be largely the result of social and behavioral-related maladaptions rather than task-related. Problems which arise outside of the work environment and personality conflicts occur in the same way as they occur in *all* work environments. However, with the advice and counsel of skilled rehabilitation personnel, such issues are usually resolved.

The CSC sponsors an annual awards ceremony honoring Outstanding Disabled Federal Employees. Formally established in October of 1968, the criterion was "exceptional job performance ... in spite of severely limiting physical factors." The finalists for this nationwide award are remarkable people. ranging from high school graduates to Ph.D.s.

They are a diverse lot of individualists, but many of them have one thing in common — they neither sought nor received any special consideration in their federal careers. Their stories encourage other disabled men and women but, more importantly, they show employers that the disabled or so-called handicapped are quite capable of performing at the highest level of efficiency. The following vignettes provide positive examples of visually impaired federal employees who were nominated for awards as Outstanding Handicapped Federal Employees.

Mr. TG — Blinded during World War II, Mr. TG began his federal service on a temporary appointment (not to exceed ninety days) as a machinist's helper with the Navy Department. In 1964, he was granted career status and promoted to mechanical parts assembler. (Annual salary approximately $9,000.)

Ms. MP — Since 1966, Ms. MP has been a dictating machine transcriber for six Army medical officers, successfully performing her job duties even though totally blind since early childhood. (Annual salary approximately $7,700.)

Mr. BP — Mr. BP has been blind since the age of five. Hired into government service in 1963 by the National Security Agency, he has progressively assumed more responsibility as a mathematician/computer programmer, even designing a special computer program to convert ADP data to braille. His program has been mass produced by IBM for use by other blind programmers. (Annual salary approximately $22,000.)

Mr. IH — Blind since birth, Mr. IH has accumulated a total of over thirty years of federal service. Hired by the Air Force as a radio and telephone repairmen, Mr. IH has developed an audio tone-producing system to replace color-coded wiring systems used in electronic repair work. He has also translated into braille all technical manuals used in radio and telephone repair work. (Annual salary approximately $12,000.)

Mr. JS — Mr. JS began losing his eyesight in 1944 while a Marine stationed in the South Pacific. Surgery was unsuccessful in restoring his sight, and, in 1961, he began his government service as a radar repairman for the Air Force. In that capacity, he repairs, modifies, and overhauls various types of electronic equipment. (Annual salary approximately $9,000.)

Mr. RW — Blinded when wounded in World War II, Mr. RW has made significant contributions to the Veterans Administration Rehabilitation Program for the Blind begun at the Hines VA Hospital. Hired in 1948, Mr. RW has continued to be the leading force in the Veterans Administration Rehabilitation Program for the Blind. (Annual salary approximately $24,200.)

Mr. KR — Born blind due to congenital glaucoma, Mr. KR accepted a position as a clerk typist trainee with the Department of Labor in 1970. (Annual salary approximately $6,600.)

Ms. AW — A blind mathematician/programmer since 1971, Ms. AW has helped to develop brailling procedures for the IBM® 360 and 370 computers used on her job at the National Security Agency, in addition to her professional work. (Annual salary approximately $12,600.)

Mr. FD — Subject to progressive deterioration of his sight due to diabetes, Mr. FD was totally blind by 1969. He was employed by the Department of Defense soon after his blindness and was promoted to a computer technician in 1972, a skill which he learned only after his blindness forced him to give up his occupation as a skilled laborer. (Annual salary approximately $8,300.)

Mr. WH — A land mine explosion permanently blinded Mr. WH while he was in military training. With a total of eighteen years of federal service, Mr. WH is presently a veterans benefit specialist with the Veterans Administration. Prior to his federal employment, he was a practicing attorney. (Annual salary approximately $13,000.)

Mr. AS — Blind by the age of eight from congenital glaucoma, Mr. AS was appointed as a computer programmer in 1968 and had progressed to a computer specialist with the Department of the Army by 1972. (Annual salary approximately $18,000.)

Ms. JY — An information receptionist with the Department of the Navy since 1971, Ms. JY was blinded at age twenty-four in an automobile accident. (Annual salary approximately $6,800.)

Ms. AL — A blind employee with the Civil Service Commission, Ms. AL has been a dictating machine transcriber for eleven years. As a member of the Missouri Federation for the Blind, the American Council of the Blind, and Real Independence Through Employment (RITE), Ms. AL has maintained an active role in community services to the blind. (Annual salary approximately $8,000.)

Mr. JM — Mr. JM lost the sight in his left eye at the age of ten when struck by a baseball while pitching; the next summer, he lost the sight in his right eye when a fence post rolled off a truck and struck him in the face. Trained as a taxpayer service representative for IRS in 1967, Mr. JM has continued to satisfactorily perform the duties of his position. (Annual salary approximately $9,900.)

Mr. OM — Blinded at the age of eight in an accident, Mr. OM has been federally employed since 1959. He began his career as a procurement analyst with the Navy and, in 1960, transferred to the Small Business Administration to assure the position of attorney. Mr. OM has received four promotions. (Annual salary approximately $28,000.)

The disabled person seeking employment used to be a small voice — usually unheeded amid the active competition of non-disabled job seekers. Even when the disabled person ultimately found gainful employment it was all too often a tawdry, backroom, out-of-sight arrangement and the work was almost invariably of the most menial sort.

The federal government, striving as always to provide leadership in employment opportunities for all Americans, has shown that the blind, as well as other severely disabled people, can function productively when they are hired based on what they have to offer, not what they have lost or might lack; when jobs are carefully analyzed to assure compatibility between job requirements and applicants' talents; when proper examining and appointing methods are utilized to facilitate placement; and when the handicapped person is not forgotten once he is on the job. The continuing record of success in this program augers well for a future in which greater numbers of disabled citizens will be able to take their proper, active places in every segment of our society and economy. When this happens, the slogan "hire the handicapped — it's good business" will have become a truism — and none will feel obliged to state so obvious a fact.

Bibliography

Department of the Treasury, Internal Revenue Service: *Report on the Washington Conference on the Employment of the Blind.* Washington, D.C., U.S. Govt Print Office, February 1969.

Oswald, Hedwig: *Blind Employees Succeeding as Job Information Specialists.* United States Civil Service Commission, BRE, Washington, D.C., U.S. Govt Print Office, October-December 1973.

President's Committee on Employment of the Handicapped: *How Federal Agencies Have Served the Handicapped.* Washington, D.C., U.S. Govt Print Office, 1972.

United States Civil Service Commission: *Employment of the Blind in Federal Service.* BRE-23, Washington, D.C., U.S. Govt Print Office, May 1973.

United States Civil Service Commission: *From Slogan to Reality: The Severely Handicapped in Federal Service.* BRE-43, Washington, D.C., U.S. Govt Print Office, February 1973.

United States Civil Service Commission: *The Outstanding Handicapped Federal Employees of the Year.* BRE-15, Washington, D.C., U.S. Govt Print Office, 1968-1973.

United States Civil Service Commission: *The Outstanding Handicapped Federal Employees of the Year.* BRE-31, Washington, D.C., U.S. Govt Print Office, April 1974.

CHAPTER 21

TECHNOLOGICAL IMPROVEMENTS IN READING MATERIALS AVAILABLE IN BRAILLE AND RECORDED FORM

CHARLES GALLOZZI

THE Division for the Blind and Physically Handicapped of the Library of Congress is responsible for the operation of a library service comparable to that offered by public libraries but with the reading matter in braille or recorded form so it can be utilized by those individuals who cannot take advantage of ordinary print because of physical impairments. With that responsibility, the division has had to plan an active role in encouraging and applying technological improvements in braille and recorded reading materials. To compensate for impairment or loss of eyesight the human system turns with increased emphasis to reading via a tactile or aural form as an effective means of obtaining information. Of all services available to blind persons because of their blindness, library service is used by more individuals than all other services combined and is generally used through the entire period of their blindness.

No other known personal reading system is as convenient, as fast, or as comprehensive as reading through normal eyesight. The past fifty years has seen an accelerating use of technology to improve those three factors in reading systems used by blind persons.

Braille was devised in France in 1824, gained official recognition there in 1854, and was introduced in America in 1860. It was the first practical method of permitting blind persons to read and to write, but compared to print it is much bulkier (about 12 to 1) and relatively slow to read (less than 100 words per minute). The first improvement came toward the end of the

240

nineteenth century. It might not be considered technological but it reduced to some extent the inconvenience of excessive bulk and it increased reading speed. It was achieved by simply assigning to certain braille characters the meanings of commonly used complete words and to other characters the meanings or values of combinations of letters which are frequent in the English language. *For, and, the* are examples of the former, being represented by a single letter; i-n-g, i-o-n, b-l-e, and c-o-n are examples of the latter. Early in the 1920s a method was developed making it possible to emboss braille on both sides of a page without the dots on one side cancelling out those on the other side. Called interpointing, this cut in half the number of sheets required for a braille book thereby cutting the bulk of a book in half.

There were no dramatic improvements in the production or reading of braille for the next forty years. Recently computers have been programmed to produce braille through inputs from punched cards, magnetic tape and disc, and from compositors' tapes. The efforts have been successful, but there is still the necessary step of fully applying known technology to eliminate the lengthy production time for braille that is a persistent problem. The storage of braille book masters in compact magnetic tape cassettes from which paper copies can be produced on demand has just become a possibility. The next two or three years may see a true revolution in braille libraries, especially if the techniques of speed-reading which are currently being applied to braille prove to be as successful as the first applications seem to indicate.

When Thomas Edison invented the phonograph he predicted its possible use as a reading medium for blind persons. In 1934 a refinement of the phonograph disc and of recording techniques made possible the use of 33 1/3 rpm records for full-length books for blind persons. Each side of a disc was made to provide fifteen minutes of reading, so that a twelve-hour novel required twenty four records. By 1958 the records could hold twenty minutes to a side, were made of unbreakable vinyl, and were half the original thickness and weight. Within the next five years the speed of 16 2/3 rpm was found to provide sufficient fidelity to permit books to be recorded. This reduced the number of records required to make up a book and made the ten-inch disc with forty-five minutes of recorded time on each side a more convenient unit. Additional refinements enabled the further reduction of playback speed to 8 1/3 rpm which is the standard today for talking books. A twelve-hour book can now be provided on four records in a lightweight plastic container. The bulk, weight, and cost of recorded books now approximate that of hardcover print books.

Another technological development of the past two or three years is the improvement of low-cost, expendable flexible records so that a full hour of recorded time can be achieved on each side of a nine-inch disc. In substantial quantities, these records can be produced inexpensively so that recorded magazines can be provided at a cost approximating their print equivalents. As a result, blind readers now receive some of their magazines directly from the manufacturer as soon as they are produced, and can keep or dispose of them as they see fit. Bulk and weight are far less than the original printed editions. The chief disadvantages of books and magazines recorded on discs is the loss of graphics and their lack of portability. Braille, like print, can be carried and read anywhere, but the disc ties a reader down to a record player which is not mobile.

In terms of convenience, the greatest technological improvement in recent years has been the development of the tape cassette and player. It has been modified so that by cutting the playback speed in half and doubling the number of sound tracks, a complete twelve-hour book can be produced on two cassettes. We now have a true "pocket book" in recorded form. Since the cassette player is completely portable, this provides the greatest convenience in reading for blind persons.

While reading by listening (175 words per minute) is faster than reading braille (100 words per minute) it is still slower than reading print with normal eyesight (350 words per minute). That problem is being attacked through speech compression. Many devices have been developed in recent years, the latest being a small, relatively low-cost unit which can be incorporated into a regular cassette player. It will permit the individual to adjust his reading speed from the average of 175 words per minute to any speed up to 500 or more words per minute, with very little loss of fidelity. The rate of 300 words per minute can be immediately utilized by most students or young persons. The higher speeds require some training to master. The same device can also be used to expand speech or any other recording. That would enable a person to take a foreign language recording and slow it down, or a music student could slow down a musical recording to be able to listen closely to every single note. Cassette players incorporating this device became commercially available in 1975.

The general public relies on the mass-produced output of printing presses and duplicating equipment for practically all of its reading except for correspondence. The braille and recorded magazines described so far are the mass-produced materials for the blind. However, they represent only a small percentage of the printed output of the world, or even of this country. Two relatively simple inventions have helped make a larger share of the printed materials available to blind persons in formats they can use — the braille writer, comparable in size and cost to a portable typewriter, and the tape recorder.

It is centuries since scribes provided the books housed in libraries or personal collections. Yet today their equivalents, volunteers, produce more books than are produced by the federal program of books for the blind. By using a braille writer a trained volunteer can produce the textbooks needed by a schoolchild or a college student, or any other work needed by a blind person but which is not popular enough to be produced in quantity by the Library of Congress. Volunteers also transcribe braille books of a specialized nature to add to the collections of libraries for the blind. Because most of the volunteers work in local communities, for local individuals, there are no statistics on their total production, but it is known that several thousand titles are thus made available each year.

The home tape recorder used by volunteers has brought an even greater supply of books to blind persons than has the braille writer. The use of a tape recorder requires less training than does a braille writer and reading by listening is more prevalent among the blind than is the reading of braille. In the twenty-five years that magnetic tape has been in use as a reading medium, it has far outstripped braille as the principal source of information and enjoyment originating in print form.

Technology is now being employed to bring together into a single, automated compilation, complete bibliographic information on all braille and recorded reading material which is available anywhere in the country, whether produced by volunteers or under government contract. All future production will also be included. This will enable any blind person to learn whether a specific title is available or how much is available on any subject or by any author, and from which sources it can be borrowed. The present service network headed by the Division for the Blind and Physically Handicapped of the Library of Congress includes more than fifty regional libraries and more than one hundred subregional libraries. It will be supplemented by the cooperation of public libraries in every community which will relay requests for information to the nearest unit in the official network. What is already a reality for a large proportion of the print-reading public in interlibrary cooperation will shortly become a reality for blind readers as well.

References

Bray, Robert S.: Library services to the blind and physically handicapped. In Kent, Allen and Lancour, Harold (Eds.): *Encyclopedia of Library and Information Science*. Vol. II. New York, Dekker, 1969, pp. 624-637.

Bray, Robert S.: Why serve them? *North Country Libraries, 11*:37-40, March-April 1968.

Clark, Leslie L.(Ed.): *Proceedings of the International Congress on Technology and Blindness*. New York, Am Foun Blind, 1963.

Cylke, Frank Kurt: Free national program to beef up services for the blind and handicapped. *American Libraries, 7*:466-467, July-August 1976.

Cylke, Frank Kurt: Planning a future of improved library services for blind and handicapped readers. In American Association of Workers for the Blind: *Blindness*. Washington, D.C., AAWB, 1973, pp. 1-5.

Gallozzi, Charles: Some effects of changes in library services for the blind and physically handicapped. In American Association of Workers for the Blind: *Blindness*. Washington, D.C., AAWB, 1972, pp. 111-115.

Gallozzi, Charles: New hope for the handicapped. *Library Journal, 92*:1417-1420, April 1, 1967.

Irvin, Robert B.: *As I Saw It.* New York, Am Foun Blind, 1955.

Koestler, Frances A.: *The Unseen Minority: A Social History of Blindness in America.* New York, McKay, 1976.

CHAPTER 22

A NEW LOOK AT THE AGING BLIND

JOSEPH KOHN

ASK any two people knowledgeable in work for the blind the number of blind people in the United States and you will probably get an argument.* The conservatives will say about 2 per 1,000 of population or 400,000 to 430,000. The high flyers will say one million or more. With so large a range, it would appear that we probably really do not know but are forecasting from particular bases.

How does this apply to the older blind? Most of us will tell you that half the blind in the United States are over sixty years of age. In New Jersey in 1972, by actual count, out of 11,000 plus names on our register 48 percent were sixty years of age or over and 60 percent were over the age of fifty.

This is hardly a new piece of information or a recent development. S. M. Green at an international meeting in 1908 in Manchester, England reported that based upon the 1900 United States census, there were 64,763 blind people in the United States and that 60 percent were over the age of fifty. Now this may be merely coincidental, but it is strange that there is such continuing consistency despite tremendous advancements in general health care, ophthalmological treatment, and prevention of blindness programs. Perhaps genetic factors are dominant here.

In our society strong support is given to educating blind youngsters and rehabilitating adults into employment. No one seems to doubt that blind children can learn and that blind adults given training can work, but what of the older blind

---

*In the United States, the usual definition of blindness is: central visual acuity of 20/200 or less in the better eye after correction, or visual acuity of more than 20/200 if there is a field defect in which the widest diameter of the visual field subtends an angle distance no greater than 20 degrees. Some states include up to 30 degrees.

person? A Princeton sociologist, Dr. Robert Scott, makes the point that because service systems concentrate on the young and the employable, adequate services are not provided to the older blind. A number of other groups and specialists agree with this and say that the most numerous among the blind are the least served. Agencies for the blind have countered with the fact that older blind people are being served through home teaching and social service units; through Medicare and Medicaid; through workshops, home industry programs, activity centers or recreational units, and the like.

In an effort to identify the needs of older blind people the Commission for the Blind in New Jersey embarked on a study supported by a grant from Seeing Eye, Inc. We visited nearly 800 blind people over the age of sixty and discussed their view of their needs. These broke down into the following:

1. *Health Needs*
   20 percent had diabetes.
   20 percent had heart conditions.
   23 percent needed dental care.
   26 percent had abnormal blood pressure.
   34 percent had foot trouble.
   34 percent had hearing problems.
   Happily 80 percent of the group reported that they were under the care of a physician or clinic. However, one out of five did not have necessary transportation, the necessary funds, or someone at home to care for them if they became ill.
2. *Housing*
   One out of three people interviewed must care for themselves and their homes and prepare their own meals. Twenty percent of the group live alone and 15 percent do not appear to be part of any family although they live as boarders. *One of the truly great problems of older blind people appears to be isolation due to lack of family interaction or lack of social information and communication.*
3. *Income*
   The vast majority of the sample studied, 80 percent, received income from Social Security, 22 percent receive

public welfare, 5 percent receive income from employment. One out of four people feel that their income is inadequate to meet basic living needs. Again a substantial number do not know how to get information about income assistance. The following are examples of this lack of information:

10 percent are not aware of income tax exemptions for blind people.

30 percent have not checked insurance policies for disability clauses.

20 percent do not receive Medicare even though eligible for it.

Most interesting, one out of four said that even if they did need financial help they would not be willing to apply for public assistance. It is not at all a new concept that blind people do not want their blindness to be synonymous with dependency and public welfare.

4. *Occupations and Activity*

Only 5 percent of the sample were receiving income from gainful employment. This is in contrast to a report from the New Jersey Department of Labor based upon a 1960 census that 29 percent of the general population over sixty were in the labor market. Although a number (15 percent) expressed interest in employment many could not travel independently, had additional disabilities, or did not have available transportation. Working at home in craft and homebound occupations seemed desirable to a number.

Based on the foregoing survey, we would strongly recommend that socialization, information, income supplements, and useful activity are the essential needs to be considered in any programs designed for the elderly blind.

References

Alpert, Helen: You can cut medical costs. *Harvest Years,* July 1971.
Belloc, N. B.: Blindness among the aged. California State Department of Public Health, Bureau of Chronic Diseases, *Public Health Reports, 71* (12):1221-1225, December 1956.

Campbell, D. R.: The rehabilitation of the blind and partially sighted. *Trans Ophthalmol Soc UK*, 77:543-551, 1957.

Donahue, Wilma and MacFarland, D. C.: Aging and blindness. In American Association of Workers for the Blind: *Blindness.* Washington, D.C., AAWB, 1964, pp. 85-98.

Hurlin, R. G.: *Committee on Operational Research.* New York, National Society for the Prevention of Blindness, 1960.

National Society for the Prevention of Blindness: *Estimated Prevalence of Blindness in the United States and in Individual States*, Publication P-617. New York, National Society for the Prevention of Blindness, 1960.

Shanas, Ethel: Financial resources of the aged: Reported resources available to those aged 65 and over in meeting medical costs up to $500. New York, Health Information Foundation, 1959.

Steiner, P. O. and Dorfman, R.: *The Economic Status of the Aged.* Berkeley, U of Cal Pr, 1957.

United States Census: Population figures. Washington, D.C., U.S. Govt Print Office, 1970.

United States Department of Commerce: *Survey of Current Business.* Department of Commerce Publication, Washington, D.C., U.S. Govt Print Office, August 1971.

CHAPTER 23

THE SUPPORTIVE ROLE OF
THE REHABILITATION TEACHER

FRANCES CRAWFORD

WHEN an individual experiences a severe visual loss, he needs to realize, as soon as possible, that living can be meaningful and satisfying without the sense of sight. A visually impaired person can become self-sufficient in caring for his daily needs and in assuming his share of responsibility for his home and family. His social and recreational activities need not be seriously limited. He can be rehabilitated through learning adaptive skills which will enable him to live effectively in his environment, to find employment if he wishes, and to make a worthwhile contribution to society.

There is a service called *rehabilitation teaching* which specializes in assisting an individual to live as fully as possible without sight in his home and community. This service, designed as a part of the rehabilitative process, exists for the purpose of enabling individuals to reach their potential for self-dependence, self-esteem, and productivity.

We know that most of our daily activities are achieved primarily through the sense of sight. We think and act in terms of "seeing." Loss of sight places severe restrictions upon the normal routine of living which are invariably accompanied by feelings of helplessness and frustration and which, in turn, contribute to personal and social inadequacy.

To cope with the traumatic effects of a visual loss, both physically and emotionally, an individual must find ways of living as a blind or visually impaired person through the substitution of other senses and the adaptation of skills in performing daily living tasks. There are compensatory techniques which can be taught to enable a person to make fuller use of his remaining senses and to live comfortably in a seeing world.

Teaching these techniques is the work of the rehabilitation teacher.

Who is eligible for this service? Rehabilitation teaching is available to adults whose visual loss is severe enough to interfere with the daily living routine and with normal means of written communication. Persons who need assistance may be located in their homes, in hospitals, and in other community settings, including facilities for the aging. Since individuals who benefit from the service differ in many respects, such as age, health, socioeconomic status, living conditions, and degree of visual loss, instruction is highly individualized to make it possible for the teacher to respond to each person in his situation and with his particular needs.

The variety of adaptive and coping skills taught by the rehabilitation teacher includes: orientation and independent movement in the home environment; personal management and daily living techniques; homemaking, home management, and household mechanics; braille, typewriting, script writing, and other communication skills; and therapeutic leisure-time activities such as hobbies, crafts, and games adapted for the blind.

Many activities, such as pouring a cup of coffee, dialing the telephone, and writing a check, require an adaptation of techniques for the person with a severe visual impairment. Instruction in many kinds of skills may be necessary if the homemaker is to perform successfully such routine tasks as preparing the family meal, cleaning the floors, and doing the household laundry. The teacher instructs in skills but also is a resource person who imparts information concerning aids and equipment and community services available to the blind and visually impaired.

The service provided by the teacher is rehabilitative in nature in that its objective is to enable individuals to achieve a maximum degree of self-sufficiency in daily living and to assume, as nearly as possible, their former role in the home and in the community. Other persons will acquire skills which lead to a vocational goal and to self-support. The rehabilitation teacher works closely with related professions and with resources in the community to assist individuals in reaching their objective.

Although individualized instruction in the skills areas is the specialty of the rehabilitation teacher, the service is much more comprehensive than the traditional type of teaching. Persons referred for instruction are likely to have experienced emotional problems related to the loss of sight which have threatened their inner well-being and which have contributed to feelings of inadequacy and loss of self-esteem. Therefore, rehabilitation teaching must be therapeutic in nature, taking into account the emotional needs of individuals, as well as their need for learning skills. Because the teacher is prepared to cope with the many problems which individuals bring to the learning situation, instruction generally can begin early with the onset of blindness. In fact, one of the most effective means of overcoming negative feelings about oneself and the loss of sight is through learning techniques which promote a sense of success and satisfaction in daily living.

As instruction proceeds, the teacher draws upon the skills of the helping professions for an understanding of the person and creates an atmosphere for learning which is warm, supportive, and free from threat. The individual who becomes adept in techniques also cultivates a more positive feeling about himself and his ability to cope with his visual loss and learns to take the initiative in resolving his own problems.

The instructional program for an individual is based upon his interest, need, and ability for learning specific skills. Medical records concerning the individual's health and physical limitations and ophthalmological information, including ability to make use of remaining vision, are necessary in planning an instructional program. The person's own evaluation of the difficulties he is experiencing in areas of daily living and communication and his desire for instruction in these areas are the chief criteria used in determining the nature and content of the individualized program. The learner is an active participant not only in planning instruction but also in evaluating his program and in setting his own goals.

Objectives which can be achieved through rehabilitation teaching may be illustrated with some brief examples:

A middle-aged homemaker, whose vision was reduced to object perception, wished to assume her responsibility again for her family and home. Under the guidance of the rehabilitation teacher, she developed skills in moving independently around her home, then learned compensatory techniques in areas of food preparation, housecleaning, and sewing and mending. Braille became useful to her for labeling cans of food, making grocery lists, and reading recipes. By regaining personal and social competencies, she felt comfortable enough to rejoin the church choir and, in time, became active again in the local PTA.

A student, who was experiencing difficulty in reading print, wished to complete his college degree. With assistance from the rehabilitation teacher he reviewed his skills on the typewriter, learned to use audio devices for reading text materials, and developed skills in braille for taking notes. Tips on grooming and selection of clothing alleviated his fears concerning his personal appearance, and campus life took on new meaning for him as he became adept in ways of initiating social contacts.

A truck driver who was forced to retire early because of his visual loss felt he was useless to himself and his family until the rehabilitation teacher helped him find ways of repairing the kitchen faucet, replacing the broken light switch, and mending the fence around his yard. With renewed confidence in his ability to cope with his loss of sight, he requested further training from the rehabilitation counselor to prepare himself for full-time employment in a new occupation.

Service to older persons in the community is of special concern to the rehabilitation teacher. Through instruction, along with other community services, many older people learn to live comfortably with limited vision and to continue independently in their own homes. Staff members of nursing homes and other community facilities for the aging are taught techniques of caring for elderly patients who are visually impaired. Individualized assistance from the rehabilitation teacher also enables some patients in hospitals and institutions to become more self-sufficient, making it possible for them to participate in foster care programs.

In this chapter I have attempted to describe the rehabilitation teaching service which is available to adults who have experienced a severe visual loss. Reaching persons who need this service requires the full cooperation of ophthalmology and rehabilitation working together to make it possible.

Individuals whose vision cannot be restored need to understand that life can have personal meaning and satisfaction as they learn to make the necessary adjustment and to find ways of living comfortably in a seeing world. As a part of the rehabilitation team, the rehabilitation teacher stands ready to assist individuals in achieving this goal.

References

Asenjo, J. Albert: *Rehabilitation Teaching for the Blind and Visually Impaired: The State of the Art, 1975.* New York, Am Foun Blind, 1975, pp. 1-79.

Crawford, Frances: Present-day concepts and practices of rehabilitation teaching. *New Outlook for the Blind,* 65(4):120-125, 1971.

Hanson, Thomas: Rehabilitation teachers — who are we? *New Outlook for the Blind,* 70(7):299-303, 1976.

Kaarlela, Ruth: Home teaching — a description. *New Outlook for the Blind,* 60(3), 1966.

Morrison, Mary: The other 128 hours a week: Teaching personal management to blind young adults. *New Outlook for the Blind,* 68(10):454-469, 1974.

Ward, Roy J.: Rehabilitation teaching. In Hardy, Richard E. and Cull, John G. (Eds.): *Social and Rehabilitation Services for the Blind.* Springfield, Thomas, 1972, pp. 350-360.

Wilson, Diana A.: Teaching multiply handicapped blind persons in a state hospital. *New Outlook for the Blind,* 69(8):337-344, 1974.

CHAPTER 24

OBSERVATIONS FROM A
PSYCHIATRIST'S PERSPECTIVE

W. Payton Kolb

In contemplating problems inherent in the various phases of work with people, I recall an old story from the archives of World War II. A psychiatrist completing a quick evaluation of a draftee asked him if he went out with girls. When the draftee replied that he did not, the somewhat uninspired psychiatrist came to life with the prospect of having discovered a potential rejectee from the standpoint of a sexual "no-no." On following this line of questioning with the obvious request for a reason he did not go out with girls, the draftee replied, "My wife won't let me."

My psychiatrist father used to tell the story on himself of the time he was exploring auditory hallucinations with a psychiatric patient. When the patient admitted that he heard voices he was asked, "Where do they come from?" To this the patient replied, "Out of other people's mouths."

To avoid as much anxiety as possible, coming from our insecurities, we try to simplify things and fit them into stereotyped patterns. The above stories point up the problems of becoming so ingrained in our work and habit patterns that we "pigeonhole" our patients and clients to the point of reducing our effectiveness.

For years we have heard the charge that ophthalmologists are an obstacle in the rehabilitation of the blind. This charge is based on the presumption that ophthalmologists are unwilling or unable to tell a patient that he is blind. Cholden has said, "The fact of blindness in their patients is extremely anxiety provoking in many ophthalmologists."[1] From personal experience I do not feel we can put the problem in such simple terms, even though there may be merit in this dynamic formulation.

There are many factors involved in the refusal of patients to accept their loss of vision. The role of the ophthalmologist is important, certainly, and our training programs are weak in preparing doctors for their role at this point in the patient's treatment and rehabilitation. Ophthalmologists are aware of this and are working to solve the overall problem.

In the same work quoted above, Cholden also has questioned, "Do counselors unconsciously perpetuate the ideal of the horror of blindness?" Although we psychiatrists sometimes contribute to these problems, we can use knowledge of human dynamics to help with the solutions.

Frequently we do not put enough emphasis on perception which is the cortical interpretation of stimuli received through the senses. When a perception is received in a highly charged emotional atmosphere it is usually distorted significantly. A patient caught up in emotions concerning the future of his vision is not in a position to perceive clearly and distinctly what is being said to him. It is important to realize the complexity of this problem.

Usually the ophthalmologist is the first person involved when a patient is confronted with blindness. The responsibility is the same if it be a neurosurgeon, family physician, internist, or some other person. The dynamics of handling the patient vary with the circumstances of the cause of the blindness such as immediate blindness due to trauma or gradual blindness from such conditions as diabetes mellitus or retinitis pigmentosa. Great sensitivity and awareness are needed in relating effectively with the patient at this time.

In psychiatry the word "dynamics" refers to the psychological and physiological components of our functioning as a psychobiological unit. When confronted with stress, certain dynamic factors come into play to protect the individual against threat and insecurity. Subsequent behavior will depend upon the degree of stress and the basic defense mechanisms within the individual. Although the alignment of the defenses will be different if the stress is sudden rather than gradual as in a deteriorating situation, the end result will be anxiety. Of the several factors involved in the resultant degree of anxiety, the personality of the individual is most important.

As a result of my experience I agree with Foulke that there is "no personality of the blind."[2] A person has a personality and a person develops blindness. In psychiatry dynamics of behavior are emphasized rather than diagnostic classification. In psychiatric illness the interest is in the precipitating stress or cause of the illness and the premorbid personality of the person before the illness.

Onset of blindness is a severe stress and is a universal stress meaning it would be a severe stress to every person. Remembering that there is "no personality of the blind," we must be aware of the personality of each person losing his sight to understand and treat the problems that occur with the onset of blindness. The direction a psychiatric illness will take is dependent principally on the premorbid personality of the individual.

The problems of how or when to tell a patient he has or is going to lose his vision can be resolved best in relation to his background personality. Usually it is not necessary to obtain a detailed past history or a complete social service work-up to understand the patient. A little extra time (of which we all have precious little), however, can mean much to the patient and his future.

Caution has to be exercised in talking with immediate families as their objectivity is greatly limited. Some accurate data can be obtained from them, but their guilt over their own fears and insecurities may make them unable to make the decisions. We all have had the experience of apprising a patient of "bad news" against the wishes of the family only to have the patient accept it adequately.

One group of definable psychiatric illnesses is known as the neuroses. These are frequently occurring illnesses with the basic component of anxiety. When the presenting symptom complex is anxiety, it is classified as an anxiety neurosis. The other classifications in this group are descriptions of the symptom complexes seen when the ego tries to resolve the anxiety. The energy is transferred to other directions and we see the depressive neurosis, conversion hysteria, phobias, and obsessive-compulsive neuroses. Blindness may precipitate a neurosis; however, the premorbid personality is the determining factor in the neurosis if it develops at all.

Although the onset of blindness will not produce a characteristic neurosis within itself, such stress almost universally will produce a reactive depression, which is usually self-limited though it may be severe for awhile. It will respond to treatment and should not be neglected. The severity, duration, and accessibility to treatment are dependent on several factors including the patient's personality, the reaction of family and friends, early life attitudes, and the attitudes of the physician and anyone else in contact with the patient.

Treatment of the neurosis as well as of the reactive depression that may develop with the onset of blindness follows the same pattern as with any person with a neurosis. This includes psychotherapy, medications, environmental manipulation, and social service with the family. Any necessity to go into the attitudes or reactions to the blindness itself should be approached firmly and honestly.

Acute psychotic episodes may occur but are relatively rare. In the presence of a severe schizoid personality, a schizophrenic reaction may occur. The same situation exists with the manic-depressive reactions; here again the treatment is the same as for anyone.

Fears of depression and possible suicide often adversely influence better judgment in handling the patient. I never have been aware of a suicide occurring as a result of the onset of blindness, though it is possible. This should not be used, however, as a rationalization for not being truthful with the patient after taking into consideration the factors already mentioned.

A major decision in management of a depressed, recently blinded patient is the selection of the best time to start an intensive rehabilitation program. Here again the basic personality of the person is the most important factor.

In general, if the training begins early in the more acute phase of depression the program needs a strong therapeutic atmosphere and a longer training period. Some patients do well with this approach and some do better to wait until some of the depression has been resolved.

Another problem to be aware of is the mental mechanism of denial which although not a disease itself can be a detriment to the rehabilitation process. We see this most frequently in a partially blind person. It occurs occasionally in a totally blind person, but most frequently in partially blind persons. This is to be distinguished from Anton's syndrome of denial of blindness associated with major cerebral lesions isolating the diencephalon from the occipital lobes.

Denial can be a valuable ego defense if used properly. If a stress is overwhelming, however, the denial can take on neurotic proportions and grossly interfere with rehabilitation. This is a valid concern regarding both the partially blind and the totally blind. There are significant considerations on both sides but we have chosen to train them together at Little Rock and we believe successfully so. We have accomplished this by individualizing the program and developing a therapeutic training milieu.

If denial is sufficiently severe then formal psychotherapy definitely can be helpful. An attitude of understanding, patience, and objectivity demonstrated by the ophthalmologist early in the process can prevent much of this problem.

Much has been written concerning patient's attitudes and their effect in all phases of blindness. As attitudes are very deepseated with many facets in the unconscious part of the mind, the control and changing of them calls forth strong conscious effort. Attitudes influence the behavior and reaction of both the worker and the client or patient.

Deeply ingrained in all of us are the fear and anxiety of blindness. This fear has come down through the ages and is given as the reason for problems in meeting blindness "head on," so to speak. It influences our behavior as described in the Cholden quotation regarding ophthalmologists and counselors given earlier. To work with a person under stress frequently produces anxiety in us with the same dynamics as described for the patient and calls for some type of control.

The emotions are more primitive than the intellect and it is important that we constantly attempt to monitor our behavior in regard to this fact. For example, some years ago a man who was deeply involved in working in the development of our center was constantly exposed to the concept that blind people can go back into the world as happy, contributing people. He intellectualized an awareness of this. Yet one day he startled us by suggesting that the center should be moved out into the country with a large acreage where the poor blind could look after a few chickens and live out their lives.

Emotional reactions are exaggerations of normal behavior and consequently we are all "ill" in varying degrees at different times. It is important then that we have some awareness of our own "shortcomings" and "blind spots" as we interrelate so closely with patients and clients and with each other. Many years ago as a young resident I was assigned the task of reviewing Dr. Norbert Wiener's book *"Cybernetics."* It seemed so technical that I can remember only that it was about guidance systems and sending men to the moon. I recall vividly, however, that in the preface, Weiner commented that the most fertile grounds for research were in the "no-man's-lands" where fields of specialization overlap. He went on to say that getting into those areas would be very difficult due to opposition from both sides. I agree with him more now than I did twenty-five years ago.

There are problems in the overlapping of the fields of psychiatry, psychology, rehabilitation, social work, theology, etc. I recently have read some of the works of Kurt Vonnegut, Jr.; in *"The Player Piano"* he has a comment that is worth study. He says, "Show me a specialist and I will show you a man who is so scared he has dug a hole for himself to hide in." Being down in a hole puts us in a position of not relating to our neighbors, consequently, we first fear and then reject.

Certainly better understanding of the fact that many things in the unconscious mind have strong influences on attitudes, motivations, and behavior is greatly needed. We may not understand why we find ourselves disliking, rejecting, fearing, loving, or feeling other emotions toward another person — colleague, patient, or client — but as Freud expressed it, "The still small voice of the intellect is the hope of mankind." This intellectual voice must be heard if we hope to accomplish the goals we have established for ourselves.

We are not master and slave, we are person and person. I recall an article in *Life* magazine a few years back concerning the controversial Baptist minister in Nashville, Tennessee, Will Campbell. This man has a unique philosophy and apparently will go anywhere to resolve problems. When asked one time how he managed to relate to various types of groups in spite of their hostility he replied, "By carrying the bedpans of their sick." When all of us become willing to do that many of our problems will be solved.

References

1. Cholden, Louis S.: *A Psychiatrist Works with Blindness.* New York, Am Foun Blind, 1958.
2. Foulke, Emerson: The personality of the blind: A non-valid concept. *New Outlook for the Blind, 66*(2), February 1972.

CHAPTER 25

PSYCHIATRIC PROBLEMS IN REHABILITATION FROM AN OPHTHALMOLOGIST'S POINT OF VIEW

JAMES L. MIMS, JR

M Y colleagues often have asked whether I am a crazy ophthalmologist who became interested in psychiatry or a psychiatrist who gained enough insight to go into ophthalmology. Seriously, my psychiatric experience has arisen as a matter of necessity and as a product of my times. As a medical student at a school with a very dynamic and active department of psychiatry, ready employment existed for students as orderlies and as senior teaching externs in a state psychopathic hospital.

Later, my internship had more than the usual emphasis on ophthalmology. During World War II, the Army unearthed my psychiatric experiences as an undergraduate and I was triphammered into a "ninety day wonder" psychiatrist. After three months of intensive training at the School of Military Neuropsychiatry, I went off to help finish the war in the Pacific theatre as a "Psychiatrist by order of the war Department."

As the war drew to an end, my soul-searching led me back to ophthalmic surgery rather than psychiatry or neurosurgery. Through the Graduate School of Medicine at Tulane University and the Tulane residency program of the New Orleans Eye, Ear, Nose and Throat Hospital, I became an ophthalmologist and in 1951 a Diplomate of the American Board of Ophthalmology. Frankly, I make no claims to being a qualified psychiatric therapist but my interest in psychiatric problems has continued, especially as they relate to dysfunction of the visual apparatus.

For many years I was a consultant in ophthalmology to the

San Antonio State Hospital where I gained much experience with neuropsychiatric disturbances as they relate to the eyes and with neuropsychiatric disturbances as a result of or in conjunction with the development of visual handicaps. During these years I also attended and studied with many patients of our local Veterans Administration Medical Service who had developed visual handicaps.

With a grandfather who had a partial visual handicap and to whom I was strongly attached, and as a result of the great rehabilitation activity after World War II, it has always seemed clear to me that rehabilitation of the visually handicapped is a normal working concern of an ophthalmologist. Somehow I did not develop the uneasiness at being around the blind that I was surprised later to find among many of my fellow ophthalmologists.

The purpose of this book is to develop a more productive relationship between ophthalmology and rehabilitation. I will discuss psychiatric problems resulting from blindness or visual handicaps from the ophthalmologist's point of view.

The ophthalmologist can well be the gateway to rehabilitation. The ophthalmologist is indeed himself a rehabilitation worker, and the first rehabilitation worker with whom the patient normally comes in contact. These concepts will be better served by care in definition.

Rehabilitation implies quite different things to individuals of different backgrounds. To me, rehabilitation is the work of restoring a disabled individual to as near normal as possible in order for that individual to become a self-reliant, self-respecting member of society as is exists at that moment in time.

If the patient (client) cannot be restored to economic productivity, then restoration to self-reliance, self-care, and self-respect are the proper business of rehabilitation. This is particularly important to those who are beyond retirement age. I reject the concept that those over retirement age who develop visual handicaps are not the proper business of rehabilitation agencies and workers.

The prefix "re," meaning again, and "habilitation," referring to going about the business of living, give a word, "rehabilitation," which means to assist an individual who has developed a handicap to reenter life. This means to live in as nearly normal a way mentally, socially, and economically as the handicap or deficit will permit.

The ultimate goal of rehabilitation is complete restoration to normal for the chronological age of the individual within the current existing society. Such total restoration of function to normal by surgery, aids, and training is, however, usually not possible given our present level of knowledge.

Thus the first step in the rehabilitation process is to establish an *inventory* of the current physical, mechanical, or physiologic capabilities of the individual.

Inventory also should be made of the patient's educational attainment or capabilities, and an evaluation of his intellectual function should be made. Psychometric testing of the visually handicapped is a science that deserves much more research and application. There are five generally accepted factors in a rehabilitation inventory:

1. Special psychological testing.
2. Medical, surgical, and optical rehabilitation possibilities.
3. Determination of a vocational goal.
4. Determination of services available for training for the above vocational goal.
5. Rehabilitation and vocational training according to individual choice (according to motivation).

We also might try to assess possible future handicap levels or the prognosis for change in the visual problem.

The ophthalmologist must quantify a medical prognosis, and the internist must similarly evaluate the general health prognosis. The complete inventory, however, must include also (1) evaluation of educational background and intellectual capabilities, (2) evaluation of aptitudes, motivations, and interests, (3) age, (4) sociological background, (5) related physical and mental disorders, (6) the functional degree of visual handicap beyond just central acuity and fields, and (7) an estimate of possible future changes in the primary disability. The ophthalmologist, being educated as a general doctor of medicine before he takes later specialty training, probably could be of more assistance in preparing this patient inventory than he usually is called upon to be. (I admit that at times educators and educational psychologists call on the ophthalmologist for more information than it is possible to give from the findings available in the usual ophthalmic examination. This sometimes is compounded by the use of psychological terms which essentially are functional descriptions without identifiable relations to anatomy or physiology.)

From this *inventory* of factors influencing the rehabilitation *goals* for a given *individual*, the *rehabilitation process* may be delineated on a logical and reasonable foundation. Reasonable decisions can be made as to which medical and surgical procedures should be encouraged, which aptitudes and attributes of the individual can be developed to substitute for the visual deficit.

Rehabilitation is accomplished by a team of medical, technical, administrative, and special services personnel building on what is left after disability has been suffered.

Since the first worker in this chain is usually an ophthalmologist, it might improve symbiosis within the team if the other members understood more intimately this very human team member called an ophthalmologist.

Consider that an ophthalmologist is one who has followed a long and strenuous educational period of twelve years or more after high school, this always has been toward one goal — the preservation or restoration of sight. He goes through the equivalent of three college educations, first a premedical student, acquiring usually a B.A. degree, then the four scholastic years leading to the M.D. degree, and, usually, the internship year which is followed finally by three to five years study as a resident physician in a specialty center. After this he often elects to endure the examinations given by the American Board of Ophthalmology, identifying him as one of approximately 10,000 Diplomates of the American Board of Ophthalmology which have been certified since 1916. Over 90 percent of the practicing ophthalmologists in the United States have followed this route voluntarily and entirely beyond the basic legal impositions of licensure as a "physician and surgeon." After all this striving to learn to help patients, it follows that the impasse of a patient who cannot be helped creates a sense of frustration and disappointment. Feelings of frustration, failure, or incompetence are unpleasant, and normal personalities withdraw from unpleasantness if possible. Many ophthalmologists, perhaps the majority, unconsciously and sometimes even consciously withdraw from the source of their feelings of inadequacy. All physicians are motivated to help their fellow beings, but soon they learn that they cannot help in the presence of some types of pathology. To survive emotionally in daily combat against death and disability, the physician soon learns he cannot let his mind dwell on a case he no longer can help, but learns it is more constructive to move on to those for whom there may be specific aid. This problem is seen to the greatest degree with the terminal cancer patient. Laymen often fail to understand the type of levity that may pervade a surgical dressing suite; this is but one way the physician preserves his personality structure against the stress of daily labors and ultimate failure against death.

A newly blinded person soon learns that many of his friends and acquaintances treat him differently — some withdraw, some deal with him in a forced euphoric manner, others become overpowering in their sympathy, several will raise their voices in conversation, while a few accomplish treating him in a normal but helpful manner. Rehabilitation personnel must understand that ophthalmologists also vary in reaction to the permanently visually handicapped and a few never make normal emotional and social adjustment to the visually handicapped, a few others react somewhat like a mother who will not give up a dying child and continue to extend help with other than medical forms of rehabilitation.

Many of the visually handicapped feel the greatest compliment that can be paid them is for a friend to obviously forget their sensory deficit. When this happens, the handicapped person has made the adjustment that must be made eventually — acceptance of the necessity to ask for help when it is needed and to accept help from a sighted person in a normal, natural manner when it is offered.

Administrative personnel for blind agencies must understand the background of the problem in getting and keeping full cooperation from many ophthalmologists. The nonmedical rehabilitation worker simply must accept without hostility the need for continuing efforts and expenses in seeking and stimulating the cooperation of the ophthalmologist. Accept the reason for his reluctance to perform always as he should and give him your understanding. Recurrently reminding and informing the ophthalmic community of the availability and *proper channels* for obtaining other rehabilitation services for his patients is a normal and necessary periodic activity of every good agency. The ophthalmologist would be more understanding, further informed, and better won to the team if he also received an initial acknowledgement from the rehabilitation agency and an occasional progress report concerning his patients.

Most private practitioners of medicine and surgery, private practitioners of ophthalmology included, share a fear, sometimes approaching paranoia, of any government agency, state or federal, having too much control over medical practice and finance. Besides his large educational investment, today's ophthalmologist has a major financial investment of $15,000 to $75,000 in ophthalmic equipment. He fears ophthalmology could become "state medicine" by the back-door route, so to speak, through a commission for the visually handicapped becoming the major economic factor in the practice of our specialty. Involvement of suitable local medical people and state societies of ophthalmology in a medical advisory board organizational pattern allays fears that a rehabilitation agency might become a bureaucratic monster.

Rehabilitation is a process of several stages. It usually begins as a relationship between a patient and an ophthalmologist. First, the ophthalmologist tries to prevent his patient from becoming a rehabilitation client, beyond the stage of medical or surgical aid. He may achieve rehabilitation by the following means:

1. Medicinal aids

2. Hygenic and environmental advice
3. Surgery
4. Optical aids

The postsurgery patient additionally may require the assistance of optical and medicinal aids, he may need these over an extended period, even for life — something many rehabilitation programs do not seem to consider. This may be stated another way — a patient may need continuing follow-up care to remain rehabilitated.

When complete restoration to the near normal state is not possible, the first psychological problems for the ophthalmologist and the patient arise. Neither the physician nor the patient finds pleasant the idea of an irreversible visual handicap. The patient with a normal personality structure will avoid the idea and the ophthalmologist is faced with the problems of (1) when he is sure and (2) when he should tell the patient he is sure of a permanent visual deficit. While there are abnormal personalities which morbidly seek a handicapped status, they are rare. Thus the crossing of the "point of realization" is initiated usually by the ophthalmologist.

Being of varied personality structures, ophthalmologists approach the problem in various ways. Some never bring the matter to the point of a positive statement. They may avoid confrontation with the attitude that eventually the problem will be solved by the patient going elsewhere. I have many times been the "elsewhere" in this scenario.

Others mount the direct frontal assault of the United States Marines and discharge their responsibility head on by telling the patient, "Well, it looks like you are blind, and there is nothing more I can do for you!"

Others let the patient gradually come to his own conclusions while they keep him busy with sometimes fruitless activity. When the patient finally asks the inevitable question, the ophthalmologist then agrees, "We've done all we can and there does not seem to be much chance of getting your sight back." There are, of course, conditions as acute optic neuritis where much return of sight can occur after a period of weeks or months, even if visual loss early in the illness is severe. Sometimes this waiting approach is the proper one.

There is also the "referral" method of handling the problem. This has the advantage of being able to say, "We sent you to the best there is. Sorry it didn't help." This involves the consultant as the one making the unpleasant judgment. Many a consultant has winced under the burden of being the first to close the door of hope.

Usually I follow a somewhat gradual approach, geared to the personality of the patient. A consultant is certainly a good safeguard, especially if the referring physician has prepared the patient for a negative result. Repetitive consultations and chasing rainbows or newspaper clippings, however, should be discouraged but not adamantly forbidden.

Too many of my colleagues feel they have discharged their responsibility when they honestly inform a patient that they no longer can help him. There are, however, at least five stages of reaction and adjustment to acute blindness that have been well outlined by George Meyer, M.D., professor of psychiatry at the University of Texas Medical School in San Antonio. The stages he describes are the following:

1. Shock and disbelief
2. Hostility and denial
3. Depression and withdrawal
4. Acceptance
5. Adjustment or adaptation

It is important to note elements of time involved in the patient's passing through these stages to acceptance and adjustment.

The ophthalmologist is bound inescapably to know and accept the often unpleasant and even occasionally dangerous reactions of the patient, reactions dangerous at times to the patient and at times to the doctor. A suicidal stage definitely must be guarded against, and the legal obligations of the ophthalmologist require careful records, the judicious use of witnesses, recording of the witnesses' observations, and the use of intraprofessional consultations.

Premature referral wastes both the patient's time and the

worker's time, and actually may result in putting off the day when the patient may willingly accept the services of the agency. Each contact worker in the initial interview situation should try to determine the readiness of the patient to accept assistance and training. Rehabilitation personnel must be aware of the various stages and attitudes that may exist along the road to acceptance, but acceptance of the existence of the disability and the need for help is essential to the effective rehabilitation. Blindness and visual handicaps, however, do not always come to normal personalities. There are some bizarre, some amusing, and some unpleasant situations where sociopaths, pathological liars, paranoid personalities, and manic-depressive psychotics develop visual loss. To those untrained or unknowing of the underlying personality problem, the reactions of the patient (client) may be misunderstood or improperly ascribed to the visual loss, and the dangers unappreciated. Agency personnel serving in contact offices in large state mental hospitals or university centers should have a background in abnormal psychology. I well recall the mental hospital patient whose cataracts I had removed without complication, and who seemed so unhappy with 20/20 vision in each eye, saying, "I can see much better with my glasses off." I finally asked her to describe what she saw without her glasses and realized for the first time that she considered her hallucinations as more clear than reality.

Rehabilitation counselors should be aware of the major psychoses, for blindness occasionally seems to aggravate and even to precipitate psychoses. Lay personnel, though, should avoid playing psychiatrist and freely call for help from trained psychiatrists, especially those who better understand the special problems associated with loss of vision.

Organic brain syndromes and cerebral arteriosclerosis of the elderly often are aggravated by associated visual loss and the accompanying spatial disorientation.

Phantom visions really do occur to nonpsychotic, otherwise nonhallucinating patients who have had a complete loss of vision (as from massive chorioretinitis) and even those who have had an eye surgically removed.

I shall never forget another mental hospital patient who was famous for his delusions of grandeur. He had generalized arthritis so severe his spine was rigid and he was quite comfortable with his head unsupported inches off the bed and with no pillow. His leg joints were fixed and he could not walk. One shoulder joint was fixed and only one clawlike hand could be brought slowly to his mouth. When I first saw him, he had completely mature or completely opaque cataracts. For a short time his vision was restored following surgery until the inflammatory process that wracked his body finally took away his sight again. During a period of lucidity he proved to have a brilliant mind and some insight, saying, "In my shape, what is there for me but my beautiful hallucinations?"

The patient's age at the onset of visual handicap and the rate of onset may modify the patient's reaction and adjustment to visual loss, but basically every previously sighted person who suffers a permanent visual loss follows the pathways I have outlined toward acceptance and adjustment, with its stages of rejection and depression and hostility before acceptance and adjustment follow.

The patient must build a new concept of his personality — of "who he is." He must establish new social relationships and often accept a different economic goal and outlook. This requires varying amounts of time and may require years for some individuals. Some never fully adjust and adapt; but, as workers for the rehabilitation of the visually handicapped, we can show understanding and help them along the road to acceptance and adaptation.

I urge the ophthalmologists to show some insight and remember their responsibility includes guiding their patients along the pathway to adjustment and adaptation to rehabilitation.

I urge the nonmedical workers to accept the ophthalmologist as he is and spend some time and money to keep reminding him how he can contribute with the rest of the team. Keep him fully informed of the pathways of referral for the patient needing rehabilitation counseling and training, and keep reinforming him at frequent intervals where this counseling and training is available. Also let him know from time to time how his patient is doing in the rehabilitation process.

References

1. Meyer, George C.: Psychodynamics of acute blindness. *Digest of Ophthalmology*, October 1971.
2. Meyer, George C.: Visual conversion reaction in children. *Psychosomatics, 10*, January-February 1969. *Psychosomatics, 10*, September-October 1973.

CHAPTER 26

PLANNING A SYSTEM OF SERVICES FOR THE BLIND

WILLIAM M. HART

A VISUAL rehabilitation center is being developed in Columbia, Missouri under the sponsorship of the Eye Research Foundation of Missouri, Inc., in affiliation with the Department of Ophthalmology of the University of Missouri. The first phase of construction is nearing completion and contains provision for clinics, laboratories, and the Lions Eye Tissue Bank. The second stage, to begin construction in one year, will provide classroom and dormitory space for the blind.

The fact that such a center is being constructed is of less importance than the philosophical base which led to its development. For this reason, the general problem of services to the blind is discussed in light of the circumstances which appear to exist at this point in time, before details of the programs and functions of the new center are elaborated.

Background for Planning

A shock wave went through the professional world of services to the blind following publication in 1970 of an article entitled "The Blindness System" by Donald A. Schon.[1] This article, which deserves to be read widely and studied intensely, speaks of the fragmentation and disorganization of services to the blind.

Simple logic advocates a well-organized system of services for the blind to provide a single point of entry for the client to a coordinated group of programs and services, and that such a system would include a pattern of financing relevant to the needs of clients. This is not, however, the situation as it exists today.

A "blindness system" does exist in this country and it is defined by Schon as an interrelated network of people, organizations, rules, and activities which include (1) all persons with severe visual impairments, (2) all agencies and groups that serve these people, (3) the training and research that affect these services, and (4) the laws and policies under which services are provided. He further states, "To call this a system is not to imply that it has defined, agreed-upon goals and coordinated programs for reaching them. In fact, the complex of institutions is fragmented and tends to behave in a disorganized way. In this sense, it is a *non-system.*"

The various public and private agencies providing assistance to the blind approximate 800 in number and are variously specialized in selected areas of service. There is little or no coordination among these agencies therefore the rehabilitation counselor is required to shop through and select from available resources on behalf of his client. The net effect of this lack of coordination is that the client has no single point of entry into the system of services and often receives incomplete or even duplicated services.

For any blindness system to function properly, the available financial resources must be relevant to existing needs of the clients. The present system, however, continues to operate on a data base which existed between 1900 and 1930. During that period the blind were identified primarily as children with the single handicap of blindness and young adults of working age. The situation today is entirely different in that it is now heavily weighted toward the aged blind, the multiply-handicapped, poor ethnic minorities, and those with significant residual vision. Nevertheless, the official blindness system continues to provide services predominantly for young adults with employment potential and children with blindness uncomplicated by other disabilities. As a consequence, only about *20 percent of the total blind population is actually being served today.*

System Design

Those who aspire to construct programs of services for the

blind must be aware of the current situation, and the reader is referred to the more complete analysis by Schon. Clearly the challenges lie in two broad areas of concern. The first of these is to design programs that have meaningful and coordinated relationships with existing efforts, and the second is to revise the criteria for application of state and federal funds. Until the latter is done, one must turn primarily to private resources for support of services in most areas of need. Admittedly, this is most difficult since private funds usually are used to supplement state resources under existing ground rules.

It is unfortunate that programs of rehabilitation have been allowed to function and grow in isolation from the mainstream of medical care. This is one of the few areas of medical concern in which this has been allowed to happen. Almost every university has a department of physical medicine and rehabilitation to provide a continuum of care for orthopedic and neurological deficits. Why should the neurological deficit of blindness be handled differently? We should have department of "ophthalmology and visual rehabilitation." Such a department should function in close coordination with the departments of physical medicine and rehabilitation since the multiply-handicapped blind now constitute a large part of the total problem. Above all, we should not let the blind become solely objects of welfare. This has not been allowed to happen with other disabilities.

The department of ophthalmology would be the point of entry into the blindness system in the university setting. The universities should provide financial support for rehabilitation of the blind and partially sighted as part of the continuum of medical care in ophthalmology just as they do for orthopedics and neurology.

There is no implication here that existing agencies are not necessary or should be disturbed. On the contrary, it is only necessary that ophthalmology become a part of the coordinated team by assuming a responsibility too long neglected. The blindness system should become the end-piece of the medical care continuum. At some point, all persons with visual loss come under the purview of the ophthalmologist. It is his obligation, in cooperation with the rehabilitation counselor, to see that his patient gets what he needs.

Assuming that it is possible to get departments of ophthalmology and their university bases to assume responsibility for visual rehabilitation in the manner indicated, there still remains the question of how all agencies in the field become coordinated. Above all there is the question of a single entry point into the system from which the client may expect automatic, fail-safe, and complete attention to his problems. There should be a telephone number which every ophthalmologist may call to set the wheels of the system in operation on behalf of his blind patient. The initiation of this process, however, does not end the role or responsibility of the ophthalmologist in the process of rehabilitation. There must be feedback in the system to the ophthalmologist which will keep him informed at all times of the progress or lack of progress of his patient. The ophthalmologist in turn must communicate his findings and recommendations which may change during his efforts to halt or reverse visual loss.

The need for a single entry point into the system may be solved by creation of a central registrar and coordinating agency for the blind and partially sighted. The responsibilities of such an agency would involve registration and referral of clients to appropriate service agencies according to individual needs, communication of information between ophthalmologists and service agencies, and acquisition of data base sufficient to establish justification of need. The central registrar and coordinating agency could be sponsored in each state by an existing state or private agency, or by a university.

In any case, each private and public agency in the state could provide some financial and program support for the central registrar and coorinating agency.

Program Design

An increasing number of states have developed rehabilitation or "adjustment centers." These centers often are state owned and operated. Some are privately owned and receive state assistance through purchase of services. A few are financed entirely with private resources. Such centers are of great value in providing curricula tailored to individual needs for acquisition of basic skills in mobility, communication, and techniques of daily living as well as assisting in career planning and reorientation. Existing centers suffer, in most instances, from isolation from medical centers, general rehabilitation programs, and other social services.

The concept of the adjustment center is valid and is here to stay, but it can be more efficient, economical, and investigative in the university setting where it interacts with and receives collateral support from programs of training, research, and medical service. Indeed, the requirements and problems of the multiply-handicapped and the aged, which constitute the increasing preponderance of the blind population, demand a medical integration. Career development problems of blind youth can be met best by the broad educational resources of the university. The need for more professional supporting and research services to the blind can be met best by the university using the facilities of a medical center.

The many interdisciplinary programs of the university are crucial to the needs of habilitation in congenital blindness and rehabilitation in acquired blindness. Not the least of these is the potential for research in a field where innovation has been modest for many years and technical equipment is strikingly simplistic in comparison to current medical and surgical developments.

There are marked differences in the needs of the congenitally blind, the aged blind, the deaf-blind, and the newly blinded of any age. No single center exists which provides for the needs in all these groups. There is a great need for special purpose centers such as those which now exist for the deaf-blind. Patient training provided in a center is only one aspect of the rehabilitation process. Many of the aged blind, for example, can be assisted best by training in their own homes and such programs apparently have been successful.

The rehabilitation center must be planned for many specific purposes. A university environment is well suited for a rehabilitation center from the standpoint of the possibility of cross fertilization with medical, educational, and research programs. Not only must the center reach out to mutualize with other resources in the university, but it must also seek to relate to existing public and private agencies outside the university.

Psychological and psychiatric studies, vocational evaluation, and career education must be extended from the university base into job experience and placement in industry and the professions. In this matter the university and its rehabilitation center has a selling job to do because the natural reluctance of employers to hire the handicapped has been accentuated by the stringent rules of the Occupational Safety Health Act.

Program in Missouri

The Board of Curators of the University of Missouri has made a commitment to support the development of a visual rehabilitation center in Columbia, Missouri. In order to facilitate this program development, the university has entered into an affiliation agreement with the Eye Research Foundation of Missouri which is a tax-exempt, not-for-profit organization. The foundation is entirely self-supporting and makes its facilities available to the department of ophthalmology for teaching, research, medical service, and rehabilitation.

The foundation owns six acres of land on which four buildings will be constructed. The first two of these are completed and opened in April 1975. They contain 14,000 square feet of space to accommodate the eye clinics, research laboratories, and the Lions Eye Tissue Bank. Two additional buildings containing 16,000 square feet of space are under construction and will provide classroom and dormitory space for the visual rehabilitation center. The four buildings are connected to each other in a quadrangular arrangement but designed to permit enlargement as the need arises.

The department of ophthalmology has the use of facilities in the University Hospital and Medical School, the clinics of the associated Veterans Administration Hospital, and those at the foundation. The department now is able to assume the responsibilities of a full spectrum of health care beginning with case finding through screening and progressing through the processes of medical care, research, training, and rehabilitation.

The facilities and programs of the visual rehabilitation center have been planned under a project development grant from the office of Rehabilitation Services of the Department of Health, Education, and Welfare.

The program which has been planned for the center is the classic curriculum of intensive training in mobility, communication skills, techniques of daily living, and physical conditioning. Vocational assessment and guidance will be provided along with psychiatric, psychological, and medical evaluation. This curriculum has proven validity and will serve as a base from which new procedures may be developed through research and continuous evaluation.

The visual rehabilitation center, unlike most other rehabilitation programs for the blind in the United States, will have the unique feature of operating within a medically oriented environment. It will serve as a teaching and research resource for the department of ophthalmology as well as for several other departments in the university. Ophthalmologists will receive needed experience in the rehabilitation of the blind and partially sighted. The departments of physical medicine and rehabilitation, education, family economics and management, psychology, and psychiatry will relate to the center in their teaching and research interests.

A cooperative program with the Department of Counseling and Personnel Services of the College of Education will facilitate the training of rehabilitation counselors for the blind. The Rusk Rehabilitation Institute will provide bed space and personnel for the multiply-handicapped blind. The Department of Bioengineering of the College of Engineering will collaborate in several areas of research and program evaluation.

There is no pretense in this development that the school of medicine is to become the nucleus of a blindness system in Missouri. On the contrary, we are seeking only to meet the rightful obligations of a state university and to cooperate in every possible way with other existing agencies in the state. The principal state agency, of course, is the Bureau for the

Blind of the Department of Welfare which has a large staff and multiple programs of services to the blind. We look to the bureau at this time for assistance in planning and later for program support.

It seems unlikely that the university or the foundation can influence directly the problem of coordination of all services to the blind. We do hope that additional forces will be brought to bear which will lead to a coordinated system in the state, and that necessary changes will occur in the allocations of state and federal funds for support of services to the blind.

References

1. Schon, D. A.: The blindness system. *New Outlook For The Blind*, *64*:169-180, June 1970. Reprinted from *The Public Interest*, (18), Winter 1970.

CHAPTER 27

THE IMPORTANCE OF A COOPERATIVE AND EFFECTIVE WORKING RELATIONSHIP BETWEEN THE COMMISSION FOR THE BLIND AND THE OPHTHALMOLOGICAL COMMUNITY

BURT RISLEY

THE Texas State Commission for the Blind has been authorized under law since 1931, but for many of its early years human services were not as much a part of our governmental life as they are today. Rehabilitation has been a state-federal program since 1920, but it was not until 1943 that federal funds became available for separate agencies for the blind engaged in rehabilitation services. Prior to 1936, only one blind person in the United States had been rehabilitated through rehabilitation programs operated under the state-federal program. Insofar as services for the blind in Texas were concerned, there was a very long period of slow growth with only very small increases in state funds from year to year and federal funds available for matching only after 1943.

During this period from 1920 until perhaps 1960 the public attitude was one which did not encourage rehabilitation of the blind, primarily because very few thought that it could be done. Therefore there were extremely limited opportunities for blind persons and practically none that would utilize their potential to its fullest extent. The potential of a blind person was most often severely limited by his undeveloped ability. This lack of development was a product of societal attitudes characterized by misunderstandings, misconceptions, a belief in superhuman senses existent in those who did manage a measure of independence, a fear of blind persons, and an errant idea that to

281

function successfully on this earth one must indeed be sighted. Today we still find the fear of blindness and loss of sight characterizing society to the extent that few people want to think about it as it might affect them personally. Of course, all of these problems have their effect on rehabilitation and present challenges to rehabilitation as we attempt to assist blind persons in overcoming the barriers placed in their path by biased and unjustified attitudes.

Since about 1960, a great deal of progress has been made in work for the blind. We are now on the way to overcoming many of the problems which beset blind persons and agencies for the blind. An important part of the aid that helped to attain what has been achieved has been the development of ophthalmology as a separate specialty of medical practice and the continually improving ability of the ophthalmological community to treat successfully conditions of the eye which in former years would have ended in irreversible blindness. Cases that formerly became blind as a result of certain conditions now in many instances either retain their sight, regain it, or retain a sufficient amount of it to function as a sighted person even though a visual impairment may be present. New procedures continually come to our attention which hold promise for individuals with visual impairments. These promising events and discoveries hold out the best possible method for rehabilitation — retaining sight. An oft used statement around our agency is the one which says, "There is no better way to rehabilitate a blind man than to restore his sight." Realizing, however, that this is possible only in a limited number of cases at the present time, it becomes imperative that the Commission for the Blind and the ophthalmological community work together to assure every client the best that both can give to assist in his rehabilitation and the best and most profitable life possible for all who may be affected by visual problems.

The first attempt at organizing a medical advisory board began in 1957. At that time the Commission had only eight district offices located in the largest metropolitan areas of the state and a single medical consultant who functioned out of

Austin. It was through this first medical consultant's efforts that approximately twelve physicians of the highest reputation from various areas of medical practice with keen interests in the field of rehabilitation were selected to make up the Commission's first medical advisory board. The medical consultant functioning out of Austin and two other ophthalmologists were included on the original board. The theory at that time was that since the Commission encountered many types of disabilities, in addition to blindness, all fields of medical practice should be represented on the board. Physicians who upheld an ardent interest in the rehabilitation of clients were retained for as long as they maintained that interest or until they asked to be relieved of the responsibility. Turnover on the board was very low and as of this date one physician originally on the board is still a member.

In 1971 it was determined that the Medical Advisory Board would be reorganized as a board consisting only of ophthalmologists. The basis for this determination lay primarily in the fact that while the Commission would serve individuals with a visual disability, the Texas Rehabilitation Commission has assumed responsibility for establishment of payment schedules for all other disabling conditions. The ophthalmologist to be included on the Board, however, would represent various areas of ophthalmology, including active practice, education, and the professional organization to which most ophthalmologists belong — the Texas Ophthalmological Association. The result, therefore, was the establishment of a medical advisory board consisting of some of the most eminent ophthalmologists in the state, as well as individuals with great interest in rehabilitation of visually disabled persons.

The reorganization of the Medical Advisory Board, as mentioned, was constituted to represent a variety of ophthalmological interest. Primary emphasis was given to representation from the Texas Ophthalmological Association. Its president, its immediate past-president, and the chairman of its insurance committee now afford ample representation on the Medical Advisory Board. In addition to those individuals, four chairmen of the departments of ophthalmology in the four existing medical schools in Texas were included as part of the reorganized board. In order to have adequate representation from each part of Texas, the state was divided into nine regions and a member was chosen from each of the nine areas to serve as a communication link between practicing ophthalmologists in that particular region, the Medical Advisory Board, and the Commission's administrators and staff. Recently, an additional member has been added to the Medical Advisory Board representing the field of pediatric ophthalmology. Since the Commission for the Blind has the original program for visually handicapped children in the nation that is completely funded from state funds, we felt it appropriate and essential to represent this emerging field of ophthalmology on the Board.

The Medical Advisory Board has three basic functions:

1. To advise the Commission, its executive officers, and its medical consultants on matters pertinent to the formulation and implementation of sound, effective, and workable departmental policies on medical services provided through the Commission in connection with the various service programs.

2. To interpret the Commission's policies on medical services to the medical profession within the state so that, through understanding of the basis and rationale of such policies, the policies might become more generally accepted, thereby promoting better cooperation between the Commission and the medical community in serving the visually disabled of Texas.

3. To serve as a forum for establishing and maintaining dialogue among all interested parties, both medical and lay, on matters pertaining to the prevention of blindness, standards of eye care, and related matters within the state of Texas and within the scope of joint concern on the part of the Commission and the medical profession.

The Commission presently has twenty-two district offices. Anytime a medical problem cannot be handled appropriately at the local level or requires policy decision, the medical problem is referred to the chairman of the Medical Advisory Board for evaluation and recommendation. The Board's legal authority is restricted to the power of making recommendations; however, since problems considered by the Medical Advisory Board are predominately medical in nature, the advice of the Board is given great weight and its recommendations are almost invariably adopted as departmental policy.

The organization of the Medical Advisory Board and the use of local medical consultants in each of our district offices results in direct contributions by at least 39 leading ophthalmologists in the state to the formulation of the Commission's policies and practices. This is approximately 7 1/2 percent of the some 537 ophthalmologists in the state of Texas. All other practicing ophthalmologists have the opportunity to and are encouraged to contribute through their regional representatives. The possibility of direct communications with the agency's staff or administration, however, most certainly is not precluded. Generally, though, issues raised through *ex parte* contact are referred back to the Medical Advisory Board for evaluation and recommendation.

One other area in which the expertise and perception of ophthalmologists in Texas are deemed vital is in identification and referral of clients to the Commission. Early identification of blindness is essential for proper treatment to be provided. The Commission is charged by legislative authority with the responsibility for maintaining a registry of blind individuals in the state of Texas. Without the cooperation received from each individual ophthalmologist, it would be impossible to even begin planning such a registry. Such a listing of blind individuals would necessitate coordination and effective rapport between the ophthalmological community and the Commission for early identification and reporting of blind individuals. However, in order to effect this coordinated plan, a liaison committee must work with the ophthalmologists to assure complete participation and consistency in reporting. This committee is the Medical Advisory Board.

The Commission's administration participates in the Medical Advisory Board meetings. Usually at least four or five central office representatives, including the Commission's executive director and assistant director, meet with the Board. These meetings are always open for input through the Board's membership or in person if some member of the ophthalmological community wishes to present his petition before the Board personally. We strive to maintain an interchange of information and ideas which results in pertinent decisions as well as an improved dialogue and understanding. In this way the Medical Advisory Board, representing all ophthalmologists in Texas, has a direct communication line to the administrative staff of the Commission. Also of significance in this interchange is the fact that representatives of the commission for the Blind can perceive any problems or difficulties that might arise and take definite action in order to preclude these problems. Such a link between the Commission and the ophthalmologists in Texas is essential to the well-being of agency clients in that they can receive, through this interchange, the best in preventive measures, diagnostic procedures, and treatment should the need arise.

We in the Commission will not be satisfied until we have arrived at a point where we can serve every blind or visually impaired person as soon as his disability becomes apparent. We are desirous of finding each of these individuals at the earliest possible moment, before the visual disability progresses or becomes permanent. Ophthalmologists are an important part of the process that will fulfill this desire. Their interest in referral at the earliest possible time is vital to the goal of this agency. At this point our funding is limited and does not permit us to carry out all the activities that we wish to in terms of services to blind and visually impaired persons in our state, but we are working hard and looking forward to the day when adequate funding will be available to meet the needs of every blind or visually impaired Texan. We utilize funding from whatever source is available in an effort to serve as many persons as possible and hopefully to make the most efficient use of each tax dollar.

It is the philosophy of this agency that if even one Texan whose sight might have been saved becomes blind, then that is one too many. It is our philosophy that if there is one person in this state with a major irreversible visual limitation who has not been provided with the specialized compensatory skills he needs in order to function as an adequate human being, then that is one too many. It is because of this philosophy that the Commission for the Blind is striving to develop the most effective and viable link possible between ophthalmologists and the agency. The importance of the Medical Advisory Board in this aspect can not be understated. With the implementation of this philosophy and making available the best in medical care and rehabilitative services, it will be possible one day to say that no Texan with a real or potential visual disability will be denied the right to develop to his maximum capabilities.

References

Cholden, Louis S.: *A Psychiatrist Works with Blindness.* New York, Am Foun Blind, 1958.

Cull, John G. and Hardy, Richard E. (Eds.): *Social and Rehabilitation Services for the Blind.* Springfield, Thomas, 1972.

Obermann, C. Esco.: *A History of Vocational Rehabilitation in America.* Minneapolis, Minnesota, Denison, 1965.

Risley, Burt L. and Hoehne, Charles W.: The vocational rehabilitation act related to the blind, the hope, the promise — and the reality. *J Rehabil, 36*:26-31.

"Texas State Commission for the Blind's Medical Advisory Board Guidelines." Unpublished, December 1970.

Wright, Beatrice.: *Physical Disability — A Psychological Approach.* New York, Har-Row, 1960.

CHAPTER 28

PRACTICAL OBSERVATIONS ON IMPROVING COMMUNICATIONS

RICHARD E. HOOVER

VERY few, if any, opthalmologists have had in-depth experience in living with, working with, training, or life planning for the broad spectrum of visually impaired or totally blind people. This lack results in a situation which Eugene Spurrier, Supervisor of the Services for the Blind and Visually Impaired, Maryland State Department of Education, has analyzed. "We find that ophthalmologists, like many other people, are simply uneducated as far as the implications (of blindness) are concerned." He further reports, "They tend to feel that these people (visually impaired and blind) are either genuises or totally dependent people who must be cared for in every way."

Mr. Spurrier related a story to me, "I was describing the vocational rehabilitation program to one of the prominent ophthalmologists in Baltimore, and he commented that all blind people either should be in workshops or allowed to remain at home and be cared for by society. I asked him if he thought I fell into either of those categories, and he indicated that I was an exception to the rule."

The collective experiences of many blind people and numerous people who work with the blind indicate that such attitudes are the rule rather than the exception.

The average ophthalmologist judges visual ability primarily in terms of distance visual acuity and how it might relate to what he thinks he personally could do with such acuity. He, therefore, tends to impose this reference, perhaps subconsciously, on his interpersonal relationships with patients, on his recommendations, and even on the inevitable forms he eventually must prepare.

On the other hand, the seeker of ocular and visual performance data as part of the other-than-medical-care and planning for an individual often expects a miracle formula from the physician regarding just what the person can see to do or what he cannot see to do. Unfortunately there is not a body of knowledge which correlates impairment of each and every aspect of visual physiology with the visual ability necessary to perform a variety of visual tasks. Until such a body of information is developed, the physician will continue to record his measurements of central visual acuity under ambient soft lighting and the worker will need to experience with each individual what can be done by residual vision. This is regardless of whether the defect is retinitis pigmentosa, primary optic atrophy, albinism nystagmus microphthalmus, aromatopsia, or countless other defects and combinations of defects. For the totally blind, there is no problem in this regard since he must at all times find other-than-visual ways of performing every task. In either case, as one very astute but nearly blind person put it, "A delicate balance must be maintained between one's ability (agility) to adapt and in turn cause people and circumstances to adapt to a point within one's reach."

Ophthalmologists must be made more knowledgeable concerning federal, state, national, international, community, and private services which are available to the severely visually impaired and blind.

The ophthalmologist wants to be assured that quality services and special attention will be brought to bear on the "unique" problems of his patient, but he is often less certain about roles and qualifications of agencies than he is of fellow neurologists, surgeons, or internists. More relevant information must be recurrently supplied to students, residents, academies, and societies on a regular basis. A one-shot program is unsatisfactory since both services and ophthalmologists are in continuous flux just as are populations and medicines. Once a physician is informed that quality services are available, he will be eager to refer his patients for such services.

The medical community should be responsible for providing to the patient, parent, counselor, trainer, employer, supervisor, etc. the visual information necessary to determine visual ability. This body of information can come only through controlled study, observation, and research and will necessarily include more than average day-time corrected visual acuity measurements for distance and, if demanded, a visual field examination which might be required for categorical purposes. Levels of color perception, accommodation, ocular motility, light and dark adaption, glare tolerance, etc. as well as standardization of measurements are often needed. Many parameters of information may be necessary to build a reasonable profile on which to predict visual ability under a variety of situations likely to be encountered by one individual. More important, the trained worker might someday be able to avoid trial and error delays as now encountered in assessing just how and why each person functions (visually) as he does when not totally blind.

One practical route is for all reporting forms in this nation to be standardized and designed to computerize answers to the basic questions such as age, sex, congenital or adventitious blindness, education, type of work performed, prognosis, and performance on standardized visual tests. There could soon be a significant mass of data available to initiate guidelines for the assessment of visual ability. Such a form, if national or even international, would eliminate the plague of myriad forms; physicians would soon learn why they are used and be less hesitant to invest time on a clearly rational form rather than wasting time filling out three or four to be put to he knows not what use.

Helpful guidance for the responsible agent (parent, teacher, counselor, etc.) in an impaired person's program or reorganization is secured by knowing what the physician has advised regarding prognosis and therapy. For example, rehabilitation workers complain of increased rehabilitation difficulties when the ophthalmologist has not been explicit concerning prognosis even when it is quite final and specific.

Clients will state that the physician did not indicate whether the vision would get better, worse, or remain static, but the worker may have a report before him clearly indicating the situation. However, if the physician has failed to discuss the problem fully with the patient, the counselor finds it difficult to develop a meaningful program. The counselor cannot be expected to give this kind of medical news to his client. It would probably destroy most working relationships between the counselor and his client and, at the same time, raise serious doubts in the patient's mind concerning the ability and integrity of his ophthalmologist.

No realistic program can be planned if the physician has left both the patient and the counselor without information upon which to plan. If a visual aid has been prescribed, the worker should know what it is, whether it is for proximal or distal use, what it purports to do, and be prepared to give supervision and training if necessary to make it effective. On the other hand, the physician may need advice from a professional worker concerning the applicability of very expensive or sophisticated devices for a particular patient; such queries should be answered with promptness, authority, and informed conviction.

Not long ago, I attended a meeting where several trainees of a blind geriatric center were asked to recount experiences which brought them to the center and their experiences and training at the center. There were, among others, two blind doctors, one severely impaired insurance executive, and a housewife who made special impact on the audience with their stories. All four seemed bitter toward the ophthalmologists. None had been told about the services available at the center by his doctor but had ferreted this out on his own or through others. All had exhausted two to five years returning to doctors for examination after examination and, as the housewife said, "getting lots of pictures and being told, 'you've got a fighting chance' but after each dilation and picture I saw less."

The insurance executive was given a visual aid at the center (after four years of visits and ophthalmic consultations) with which he felt he was able to return to a productive executive position. The doctors both indicated that an earlier introduction of the rehabilitation process would have allowed them to change course and salvage some professional ties and productivity which were lost because of elapse of time and contacts. The point is that a doctor should not be expected to know all about blindness and available services if he encounters only one or two such in his career — just as most current ophthalmologists do not undertake modern day vitreous surgery — but just as the ophthalmologist usually knows how and where to refer for consideration of vitreous surgery, the physician should know or find out how and where to refer for visual and blind rehabilitation. This assures greater and more meaningful communication between the ophthalmologist and the specialists who must prepare, teach, and supervise the growth, education, and social and vocational endeavors of the visually impaired and totally blind.

As a practical test, how many ophthalmologists know the whereabouts of, organization of, and services available from the six largest national agencies?

The American Foundation for the Blind
The National Industries for the Blind
The National Council of State Agencies for the Blind, Etc.
The National Federation for the Blind
The National Accreditation Council for Agencies Serving the Blind and Visually Handicapped
The American Printing House for the Blind

This list could be enlarged many times. There is a need also to know local services and specific considerations for the patient in work opportunities, tax exemptions, transportation, education, etc. This should be furnished on a current basis or at least once a year by local agencies to the ophthalmic community thus keeping each well informed about the other. As a practical matter, such simple mechanisms for communications have worked poorly in the past for the rather embarrassing reason that the average doctor is not committed to and is sometimes ignorant of the needs of his patients who have lost vision and have no hope of restoration. The ophthalmologist generally has not been prepared to encompass rehabilitation as part of an individual's medical therapy. This preparation should take place early in residency training and should be a requirement of all our 161 programs. He would transfer this knowledge and these attitudes to his nurses, technicians, and secretaries and thus enhance smooth and useful communications between the physician, his medical co-workers, and those concerned with the rehabilitation of any individual patient or group of patients.

Summary

1. The ophthalmologist must be prepared to envision rehabilitation as part of medical therapy during his early training.

2. He must also be prepared to furnish rehabilitation workers with visual data about a patient in enough depth to lay a foundation for estimating visual ability.

3. He should know when and how to communicate to a patient the need for services and information without unnecessary delay.

4. He should know where and how to refer for such services.

5. The rehabilitation workers should communicate to the ophthalmologist their capacity and potential to supply needed services.

6. The people responsible for rehabilitation should assume leadership in standardization of forms and accumulation of data.

7. The rehabilitation specialist should communicate to the ophthalmologist the services available on a federal, state, community, and private level.

8. The rehabilitation specialist should take a leading role in the organization of information and training courses for residents in the training programs.

9. The rehabilitation specialist must communicate his competency to the physician in a specific way — both as to potential and end results, e.g. if a visual aid has been prescribed, does the worker understand its purpose, can he train or supervise its use?

10. Progress reports to the physician from the worker are

needed to enable the physician to assess the efficiency of the process and continue his interest in his patient and in rehabilitation.

NAME INDEX

SUBJECT INDEX

A

Abetalipoproteinemia, 36
Abortion laws, 36
Acceptance of blindness, 120, 226
Access to information, client's right of, 182-183
Accountability, 6-8
Acute psychotic episodes, 258
Adjustment centers (*See* Rehabilitation centers)
Adjustment to blindness (*See* Blindness)
Adjustment training, 14
Adult children of visually impaired aged, 89
Adult onset of glaucoma, 23
Advanced glaucoma, 85
Advice about work opportunities, 224-228
Advocacy services
  blind consumer's right to, 178
  defined, 178
Age at onset of blindness, 271
Aging, enzymatic alteration of, 27
Aging blind, 15-16, 89, 246-249, 277
  activities of, 248
  health needs, 247
  housing needs, 247
  inadequacy of services for, 247
  income needs, 247-248
  needs of, 247-248
  number of, 246
  occupations, 248
  rehabilitative teaching, 253
Albinism, 33, 76
  ocular, 35
Alkaptonuria, 33
Ambient devices, 57
American Association of Workers for the Blind, 194
American Foundation for the Blind, Inc., 74, 87
American Printing House for the Blind, 169
American Printing House Quota, 211
Amniocentesis, 34
Amniotic fluid or cells
  direct analysis of, 34-35
  indirect analysis, 35
Anatomical orientation, 117
Anesthesias, 114
Angle closure glaucoma, 23
Aniridia, 30
Antimetabolites, 27
Anton's syndrome of denial of blindness, 259
Anxiety, 257, 259
Anxiety neurosis, 257
Aphonia, 114
Appeals process, 177-179
Appreciation spectrum, 219-220
Aptitude tests, 170
Archie Bunkerism, 198
Architectural barriers, 145
Arkansas Enterprises for the Blind, 233-234
Artificial eye, 91-92
Asphenic lens surfaces, 22
Asphenic lenses, 79
Attitudes, 259
  concreteness of expression, 202-203
  counseling to change, 200-201
  counselor's, 201-203
  defined, 191-193
  direct educational programs, 199
  dynamic functions of, 203
  empathy, 202
  environmental change, 200
  false generalization, 198
  fear, 196
  general inclusion, principle of, 199
  genuineness, 202
  intergroup contact or interaction, 199
  legislative change, 200
  modification of, 199-201

299

Physical arrangements, 204-205
Physical contact, 205
Physical limitations of work setting, 145
Physical restoration, 13-14
Physical therapy, 172
Physicists, 13
Physiological satisfaction need, 153
"Pigeonholing" of patients, 255
Pity for blind, 197
Placement of jobs (*See* Vocational placement)
"The Plague," 85
Planning a system of services for the blind, 273-280
background for, 273-274
central registrar and coordinating agency, 276
defined, 274
design of program, 276-278
design of system, 274-276
Missouri program, 278-280
rehabilitation centers, 276-278
scope of system, 274
Playboy, 207
The Player Piano, 260
Point mutations, 30
Point of realization, 268
Political campaigns, challenges to, 3
Positive regard, attitude of, 202
Post-employment services, 14
Potential devices of use to blind, 49
Precision equipment, 50
Prejudice against blind, 197-198
clusters, 198
factors associated with, 197-198
individual personality, 197
socioeconomic status, 197
Preliminary counseling sessions, 118
Premorbid personality, 257-258
Prenatal detection, 34-35
Prevocational training, 14
Prism binoculars, 78
Prism monoculars, 78
Problems of the blind, 45-48
Professional differences, problems created by, 211
Professional education, 89
Professional placement, 146-147
long-range planning for, 147
Professional rehabilitation workers

attitudinal considerations of, 189-208
(*See also* Attitudes)
considerations of, 206-207
counseling considerations, 189-191
requirements of, 189
techniques of (*See* Counseling techniques)
Prognostic advances, 25-26
Projection as defense mechanism, 124
Projective personality tests, 170
Proliferative diabetic retinopathy, 66, 68, 71
Prompt decision making and services, right to, 183
Psychiatric illness, 257
Psychiatric problems in rehabilitation, 262-272
Psychiatrists, 13
Psychiatrists' perspective, 255-261
Psychological adjustment curve, 189-190
Psychological adjustment to blindness, 114-115, 189-191
Psychological effects of disabilities, 116-117
Psychological tests used with blind persons, 168-170
Psychometric testing, 264
Psychoses, 270
Psychosomatic medicine, 114-115
Psychotherapy, 172, 258-259
attitudinal change through, 200-201
Public awareness, 89
Public Law 89-565, 143
Public Law 93-112, 180
Public Law 113, 12
Pygmalion effect, 194

R

Radical surgical excisions, 25
Radio Information Center for the Blind (Philadelphia, Pennsylvania), 207
Radio spots, 89
Radio technicians, 13
Radioimmune diagnosis, 27
Radioisotope therapy, 27
Rap sessions, 88
Rate of onset of blindness, 271
Rationalization as defense mechanism, 123-124